SORANUS'

GYNECOLOGY

SORANUS'

TRANSLATED WITH AN INTRODUCTION BY

OWSEI TEMKIN, M.D.

THE JOHNS HOPKINS UNIVERSITY PRESS

BALTIMORE AND LONDON

GYNECOLOGY

WITH THE ASSISTANCE OF

Nicholson J. Eastman, M.D.

Ludwig Edelstein, PH.D.

AND *Alan F. Guttmacher,* M.D.

© 1956 by The Johns Hopkins Press, Baltimore
All rights reserved
Printed in the United States of America on acid-free paper

Johns Hopkins Paperbacks edition, 1991
4 6 8 9 7 5 3

The Johns Hopkins University Press
2715 North Charles Street
Baltimore, Maryland 21218-4363
www.press.jhu.edu

Library of Congress Cataloging-in-Publication Data

Soranus, of Ephesus.
[Gynaecia. English]
Soranus' gynecology/translated with an introduction by Owsei
Temkin: with the assistance of Nicholson J. Eastman, Ludwig
Edelstein, and Alan F. Guttmacher.—Softshell Books ed.
p. cm.
Translation of: Gynaecia.
Reprint. Originally published: Baltimore: Johns Hopkins Press.
© 1956
Includes bibliographical references and index.
ISBN 0-8018-4320-0 (pbk. : alk. paper)
1. Medicine, Greek and Roman. 2. Gynecology I. Temkin, Owsei,
1902- . II. Title.
[DNLM: WZ 290 S713g 1956a]
R126.S623 1991
618. 1—dc20
DNLM/DLC
for Library of Congress 91-20791

A catalog record for this book is available from the British Library.

TO THE MEMORY OF

JOHANNES ILBERG

(1860–1930)

on whose edition of the Greek text
this translation is based

PREFACE

This English translation of Soranus' *Gynecology* owes its origin to the initiative of Dr. Nicholson J. Eastman, Professor of Obstetrics and Director of the Department of Obstetrics at the Johns Hopkins University. Nearly twenty years ago our group, comprising Dr. Eastman, Dr. Alan F. Guttmacher, now Clinical Professor of Obstetrics and Gynecology at the College of Physicians and Surgeons and Director of Obstetrics and Gynecology at the Mount Sinai Hospital, New York, Dr. Ludwig Edelstein, now Professor of Humanistic Studies at the Johns Hopkins University, and I began to meet twice weekly at the Institute of the History of Medicine of the Johns Hopkins University. At these informal meetings I submitted the draft of a translation which was read, discussed, and greatly changed. Dr. Eastman and Dr. Guttmacher gave of their professional medical knowledge and stylistic skill, while Dr. Edelstein, as a classical scholar, watched over the linguistic aspect. Thus, in the course of seven years, the translation was completed. The war interrupted the necessary task of revision, which could not be resumed before 1946. In 1949, Dr. I. E. Drabkin made available to me his edition of the *Gynaecia* of Caelius Aurelianus (see below, p. xliv) which proved helpful in elucidating several passages. To Dr. Drabkin as well as to the several scholars who occasionally attended our meetings and made valuable suggestions I am greatly indebted. The revised manuscript has been submitted to the three other members of the group, and Dr. Edelstein, in particular, has gone to great pains in pointing out doubtful passages and advising me on interpretation. However, the responsibility for final decisions and, therefore, for all shortcomings rests upon me alone.

We have tried to keep the translation as close to the Greek text as possible, even when the meaning seemed unclear to us. For this reason, we have also avoided undue use of modern medical terminology and of forced interpretations in the light of present-day knowledge. Throughout, it was our purpose to acquaint the reader with the reasoning, clinical experience, and imagery of an ancient physician whose outlook and background were very different from our own.

The Introduction as well as the comments have been kept very brief, since the details and background of ancient gynecology can be found in such works as McKay's *History of Ancient Gynecology* (New York, William Wood, 1901); Fasbender's *Geschichte der Geburtshülfe* (Jena, 1906); Ricci's *Genealogy of Gynaecology* (2nd edition, Philadelphia, Blakiston, 1950); and Diepgen's *Die Frauenheilkunde der alten Welt* (München, 1937).

The list of names is intended as a means of quick orientation; it is chiefly based on the biographies in Pauly-Wissowa's *Real-Encyclopädie der classischen Altertumswissenschaft*. The index for the materia medica lists the drugs and foods according to their popular English names. The identification of ancient botanical terms is notoriously difficult, especially when, as in Soranus' *Gynecology*, no descriptive details are given. Apart from Liddell and Scott's *Greek-English Lexicon*, I have mainly relied upon Goodyer's translation of Dioscorides (in the edition by Gunther); Sir

Arthur Hort's translation of Theophrastus' *Enquiry into Plants;* Francis Adams' translation of Paulus of Aegina; Spencer's translation of Celsus; and above all, on the comments by Berendes in his *Des Pedanios Dioskurides aus Anazarbos Arzneimittellehre.* Exactness of nomenclature would have been misleading, and the popular English names seemed to correspond much better to Soranus' own usage.

I wish to express my personal gratitude to my wife, who has helped me in all stages of the preparation of this work.

The assistance of Miss Virginia Davidson, Miss Elise Moale, and Mrs. Janet Koudelka in the preparation of the manuscript is gratefully acknowledged.

Owsei Temkin, M.D.

THE JOHNS HOPKINS UNIVERSITY
INSTITUTE OF THE HISTORY OF MEDICINE
July, 1955

CONTENTS

* Angular brackets < > around chapter headings denote that the heading and possibly parts of the chapter are missing. Addition of the word *missing* indicates that the chapter is entirely lacking.

LIST OF ILLUSTRATIONS

BIBLIOGRAPHICAL ABBREVIATIONS

Alexander of Tralles, ed. Puschmann: *Alexander von Tralles.* Original-Text und Übersetzung nebst einer einleitenden Abhandlung. Ein Beitrag zur Geschichte der Medicin von Theodor Puschmann. 2 vols. Wien, W. Braumüller, 1878–1879.

Anonymus Londinensis, ed. Jones: *The Medical Writings of Anonymus Londinensis.* By W. H. S. Jones. Cambridge, University Press, 1947.

Aretaeus (Adams' translation): *The Extant Works of Aretaeus, the Cappadocian.* Edited and translated by Francis Adams. London, 1856 (The Sydenham Society).

Aristotle, *Oxford transl.: The Works of Aristotle.* Translated into English under the editorship of W. D. Ross. Oxford, The Clarendon Press.

"Hist. animal.": Historia animalium, by D'Arcy Wentworth Thompson, vol. IV, 1910.

"De gener. animal.": De generatione animalium, by Arthur Platt, vol. V, 1912.

"Politica," by Benjamin Jowett, vol. X, 1921.

Barbour (1914): A. H. F. Barbour, Soranus on Gynaecological Anatomy, *Seventh International Congress of Medicine,* London, 1913. Section XXIII, History of Medicine, London, 1914, pp. 269–283.

Berendes: *Des Pedanios Dioskurides aus Anazarbos Arzneimittellehre in fünf Büchern.* Übersetzt und mit Erklärungen versehen von J. Berendes. Stuttgart, F. Enke, 1902.

Caelius Aurelianus, *Acute Dis.*
Caelius Aurelianus, *Chronic Dis.* } :

Caelius Aurelianus, *On Acute Diseases* and *On Chronic Diseases.* Edited and translated by I. E. Drabkin. The University of Chicago Press, 1950.

Caelius Aurelianus, *Gynaecia:* Caelius Aurelianus, *Gynaecia.* Fragments of a Latin version of Soranus' *Gynaecia* from a thirteenth century manuscript. Edited by Miriam F. Drabkin and Israel E. Drabkin. Baltimore, The Johns Hopkins Press, 1951 (*Supplements to the Bulletin of the History of Medicine,* 13).

Celsus: *Celsus, De medicina.* With an English translation by W. G. Spencer. 3 vols. (Loeb Classical Library).

Deichgräber, *Empirikerschule:* Karl Deichgräber, *Die griechische Empirikerschule.* Sammlung der Fragmente und Darstellung der Lehre. Berlin, Weidmann, 1930.

Diepgen: Paul Diepgen, *Die Frauenheilkunde der alten Welt.* München, J. F. Bergmann, 1937 (*Handbuch der Gynäkologie,* herausgegeben von W. Stoeckel, 12. Bd., 1. Teil).

Dioscorides: *Pedanii Dioscuridis Anazarbei De materia medica libri quinque.* Edidit Max Wellmann. 3 vols. Berolini, Weidmann, 1907–1914.

Ermerins: *Sorani Ephesii liber de muliebribus affectionibus.* Recensuit et Latine interpretatus est Franciscus Zacharias Ermerins. Traiecti ad Rhenum, 1869.

Fasbender, *Entwickelungslehre:* Heinrich Fasbender, *Entwickelungslehre, Geburtshülfe und Gynäkologie in den hippokratischen Schriften.* Stuttgart, Ferdinand Enke, 1897.

Fasbender, *Geschichte:* Heinrich Fasbender, *Geschichte der Geburtshülfe.* Jena, Gustav Fischer, 1906.

Freeman, *Ancilla:* Kathleen Freeman, *Ancilla to the Pre-Socratic Philosophers.* Cambridge, Harvard University Press, 1948.

Galen, ed. Kühn: *Claudii Galeni Opera omnia.* Editionem curavit Carolus Gottlob Kühn, 20 vols. Lipsiae, 1821–1833.

Galen, *On the Natural Faculties:* (same title) with an English translation by Arthur John Brock (Loeb Classical Library).

Galen, *De usu partium: Galeni De usu partium libri XVII.* Recensuit Georgius Helmreich. 2 vols. Lipsiae, Teubner, 1907–1909.

Gunther: *The Greek Herbal of Dioscorides,* Illustrated by a Byzantine A.D. 512. Englished by John Goodyer A.D. 1655, edited and first printed A.D. 1933 by Robert T. Gunther. Oxford, University Press, 1934.

Hippocrates, ed. Jones: *Hippocrates.* With an English translation by W. H. S. Jones. 4 vols. (Loeb Classical Library). [Vol. 3 transl. E. T. Withington].

Hippocrates, ed. Littré: *Oeuvres complètes d'Hippocrate.* Traduction nouvelle avec le texte Grec en regard . . . par E. Littré. 10 vols. Paris, J. B. Baillière, 1839–1861.

Ilberg: *Sorani gynaeciorum libri IV* etc. Edidit Ioannes Ilberg. Lipsiae et Berolini, Teubner, 1927 (*Corpus medicorum Graecorum,* IV).

Ilberg, *Überlieferung: Die Überlieferung der Gynäkologie des Soranus von Ephesos,* von Johannes Ilberg. Leipzig, Teubner, 1910 (Abhdlg. d. philol.-hist. Klasse d. königl. sächsischen Gesellsch. d. Wissenschaften, No. II).

Kind in *Pauly-Wissowa:* Article "Soranus" by Ernst Kind in *Pauly-Wissowa,* zweite Reihe, dritter Band, cols. 1113–1130.

Lesky: Erna Lesky, *Die Zeugungs- und Vererbungslehren der Antike und ihr Nachwirken.* Wiesbaden, 1951 (Akademie der Wissenschaften und der Literatur, Abhdlg. d. geistes- und sozialwissenschaftlichen Klasse, Jahrgang 1950, Nr. 19).

Liddell and Scott: *A Greek-English Lexicon* compiled by H. G. Liddell and R. Scott. A new edition revised and augmented throughout by Henry Stuart Jones. Oxford, Clarendon Press, 1925–1940.

Lüneburg: *Die Gynäkologie des Soranus von Ephesus.* Übersetzt von H. Lüneburg. Commentirt und mit Beilagen versehen von J. Ch. Huber. München, J. F. Lehmann, 1894 (Bibliothek medicinischer Klassiker, I).

Muscio: *see* Rose.

Oribasius, *Collect. med.:* Oribasius, "Collectiones medicae," in: *Oeuvres d'Oribase,* texte grec . . . traduit . . . par Bussemaker et Daremberg. 6 vols. Paris, 1851–1876.

Partington: J. R. Partington, *Origins and Development of Applied Chemistry.* London, New York, Toronto, Longmans, Green and Co., 1935.

Paul of Aegina (Adams' translation): *The Seven Books of Paulus Aeginata.* Translated from the Greek with a Commentary . . . by Francis Adams. 3 vols. London, 1844–1847 (The Sydenham Society).

Pauly-Wissowa: Paulys Real-Encyclopädie der classischen Altertumswissenschaft. Neue Bearbeitung herausgegeben von Georg Wissowa. Stuttgart, J. B. Metzler, 1894–.

Pliny: *Pliny, Natural History.* With an English translation in ten volumes (Loeb Classical Library). Of the volumes published so far, vols. I–V and IX are translated by H. Rackham, vol. VI by W. H. S. Jones.

Rose: *Sorani gynaeciorum vetus translatio Latina* nunc primum edita cum additis Graeci textus reliquiis a Dietzio repertis atque ad ipsum codicem Parisiensem nunc recognitis a Valentino Rose. Lipsiae, Teubner, 1882.

Rose, *Anecdota:* Valentin Rose, *Anecdota Graeca et Graecolatina.* 2 vols. Berlin, Ferdinand Duemmler, 1864–1870.

Singer: Charles Singer, *The Earliest Chemical Industry.* London, The Folio Society, 1948.

Theophrastus, *Hist. plant.:* Theophrastus, *Enquiry into Plants.* With an English translation by Sir Arthur Hort. 2 vols. (Loeb Classical Library).

Wellmann, *Fragmente:* Max Wellmann, *Die Fragmente der sikelischen Ärzte,* Akron, Philistion und des Diokles von Karystos. Berlin, Weidmann, 1901.

INTRODUCTION

Soranus was one of the most learned, critical, and lucid authors of antiquity. But, though his name attained great fame, we know little of the circumstances of his life, and most of his writings have been lost.[1] He was born at Ephesus, a city in Asia Minor, the son of Menandrus and his wife, Phoebe, probably in the second half of the first century A.D. According to his biographer, Suidas,[2] he studied in Alexandria, still the great center of scientific medicine. Like so many Greek physicians, Soranus eventually turned to Rome where he practiced medicine at the time of the emperors Trajan (98–117) and Hadrian (117–138). He thus belongs to the early second century and died at about the time when Galen was born.

Nearly twenty works have Soranus as their author.[3] Of those preserved in the original Greek, the *Gynecology* is the most important. There are also extant in Greek [4] short treatises "On Bandages" and "On Fractures," the latter possibly part of the lost "Surgery," as well as a "Life of Hippocrates"

[1] For a critical discussion of Soranus' life and writings see the article by Ernst Kind in *Pauly-Wissowa,* s.v. "Soranus."

[2] Suidas, *Lexicon,* ed. Ada Adler, Leipzig, 1928–1938, s.v. "Soranus." Suidas lists two physicians under the name of Soranus. However, their identity has been generally accepted.

[3] Kind in *Pauly-Wissowa.*

[4] The Greek writings preserved have all been edited by Ilberg in vol. IV of the *Corpus Medicorum Graecorum* (see below).

ascribed to Soranus.[5] Another major work, *On Acute and Chronic Diseases,* has come down to us in the Latin paraphrase of Caelius Aurelianus who lived in the fifth or sixth century.[6] Caelius Aurelianus' paraphrase can to all practical purposes be considered a translation of Soranus' Greek original.

Viewing Soranus' writings as a whole, we can say that they ranged over a wide field of biological and medical science. Not only did he deal with gynecology, internal medicine, surgery, materia medica, hygiene, ophthalmology, medical history, and anatomical nomenclature, but he also included treatises on embryology and on the soul among his works. His influence on following generations was correspondingly broad. The Church father, Tertullian, esteemed him highly for his acquaintance with the tenets of other philosophers and for his view of the soul as a corporeal substance, although he deplored the fact that Soranus had "defrauded (the soul) of its immortality." [7] St. Augustine called Soranus "medicinae auctor nobilissimus"; John of Salisbury mentioned him on a par with Socrates, Plato, Aristotle, and Seneca.[8] Others made extensive use of his etymological explanations of anatomical terms and his references to the opinions of preceding physi-

5 Opinion is divided as to whether this vita is a fragment from Soranus' large work, "Lives of Physicians, Sects, and Treatises" (Kind, *loc. cit.* col. 1115), or erroneously ascribed to him (cf. Edelstein, article "Hippocrates," *Pauly-Wissowa,* Supplementband VI, col. 1294 ff.).

6 Caelius Aurelianus has transmitted to us 3 books, "Celerum sive acutarum passionum" (to which Soranus refers in the *Gynecology,* books III, 25 and IV, 6 (below, pp. 148, 183), and 5 books, "Tardarum sive chronicarum passionum." Both works are now easily accessible in I. E. Drabkin's edition and translation.

7 On Soranus and Tertullian see Heinrich Karpp in *Zeitschrift für die neutestamentliche Wissenschaft und die Kunde der älteren Kirche* 1934, vol. 33, pp. 31–47.

8 See Hermann Usener, *Kleine Schriften,* vol. 3, Leipzig-Berlin, 1914, p. 32.

cians.[9] But his chief fame rested on two circumstances. In the first place, he became recognized as the most outstanding representative of the methodist sect. It is impossible to understand Soranus outside the framework of this particular school of ancient medicine, while at the same time our knowledge of the methodist sect would remain scanty without the help of Soranus' work. Second, his *Gynecology* represented ancient gynecological and obstetrical practice at its height. Through the work of translators, abbreviators, and compilers, much of Soranus' views and practices survived through the middle ages into the sixteenth century.

The Methodist Sect

Ancient Graeco-Roman medicine never achieved the unanimity as to method and facts which might have made it a universally accepted progressive science. The Hippocratic collection, far from being the work of one author, shows a wide diversity of views among the physicians who lived and wrote around 400 B.C. In the third century B.C. there emerged two main theoretical schools, or sects, sharply divided by philosophical and scientific differences, although by no means united in themselves. The so-called "dogmatic" sect believed in the necessity and possibility of rational scientific investigation as the basis of medicine. Since many of the causes of diseases were "hidden," they had to be unveiled by anatomical dissection and experiment, so that diseases might be explained and their treatment guided by rational arguments. The great anatomists, Herophilus and Erasistratus, both of whom worked in Alexandria in the third century B.C., were out-

[9] See Kind in *Pauly-Wissowa,* and Werner Jaeger, *Diokles von Karystos,* Berlin, 1938, p. 190 ff.

standing representatives of this sect. But probably even during their lifetime, the "empirical" sect arose in opposition. The empiricists denied that nature was comprehensible and therefore rejected the investigation into "hidden causes" of disease. Instead, as their name indicated, they made experience their main principle. Guided by his own accumulated experience as well as by that of other reliable practitioners, the physician would recognize such "evident" causes as hunger, cold, etc., would diagnose a disease according to its symptoms, and would know the treatment that had proved efficient in these cases. Only where confronted by a new disease might he reason by analogy from the known.

The sects of dogmatists and empiricists had both originated in Alexandria. In contrast, the third and youngest sect, that of the "methodists," though the product of Greek physicians, developed in Rome. Here, in the first century B.C., Asclepiades of Prusa, a city of Bithynia, settled as a successful orator and physician. He elaborated a medical theory akin to the philosophical speculations of Epicurean atomism. The body, an aggregate of ever-moving atoms, was transversed by pores carrying body fluids and pneuma. Health and disease depended upon the size, shape, number, and movement of the particles, and the condition of the pores and their contents.[10] In conformity with this physical theory of the organism, Asclepiades emphasized physicotherapy. While all sects considered a proper regimen the most important factor in the treatment of internal diseases, Asclepiades insisted on moderation in the use of food or wine, and on massage, walking, and passive exercise, cold water, and bathing.[11]

[10] See Caelius Aurelianus, *Acute Dis.* I, ch. 14.

[11] Pliny XXVI, 3. On the system of Asclepiades as well as for the following see Meyer-Steineg, *Das medizinische System der Methodiker,* Jena, 1916

The next step was made by his pupil Themison, about whose life and intellectual development we are but badly informed. But it seems that at some time Themison began to deviate from the teachings of his master Asclepiades. He established the doctrine of the "communities," i.e. a few general conditions common to large numbers of diseases. Besides, in his therapy he paid attention to the stages of the disease. There is some probability that the work of Celsus reflects in some respects the doctrines of Themison.[12]

Although Themison was not the founder of the methodist sect, he certainly laid the basis for its rise, in the early part of the first century A.D., as a rival of the older dogmatic and empirical sects.[13] Thessalus, the much maligned physician of the Emperor Nero (54–68 A.D.), appears as its outstanding leader.

Philosophically, the main difference between the methodists and the other sects was their rejection of both etiological research and mere experience. Possibly under the influence of Pyrrhonean scepticism,[14] they did not believe in the necessity of inquiring into the causes of disease, and disparaged anatomy and physiology, as well as humoral pathology. On the other hand, they thought that the physician needed a more secure knowledge than was offered by experience. This knowl-

(Jenaer medizin-historische Beiträge, H. 7–8); T. Clifford Allbutt, *Greek Medicine in Rome,* London, 1921. Ludwig Edelstein, Article "Methodiker," in *Pauly-Wissowa,* Supplementband VI, cols. 358–73; I. E. Drabkin, Soranus and His System of Medicine, *Bull. Hist. Med.* 1951, vol. 25, pp. 503–18, and the Introduction to his edition of Caelius Aurelianus, *On Acute Diseases* and *On Chronic Diseases.*

12 Owsei Temkin, Celsus' "On Medicine" and the Ancient Medical Sects, *Bull. Hist. Med.* 1935, vol. 3, pp. 249–64.

13 Ludwig Edelstein, Article "Methodiker," in *Pauly-Wissowa,* Supplementband VI, cols. 358–73.

14 Edelstein, *ibid.*

edge could be derived from the phenomena of the diseases themselves. The basic tenets of the methodists are best summarized in the following statement of Celsus.

> . . . certain physicians of our time, following, as they would have it appear, the authority of Themison, contend that there is no cause whatever, the knowledge of which has any bearing on treatment: they hold that it is sufficient to observe certain general characteristics of diseases; that of these there are three classes, one a constriction, another a flux, the third a mixture. For the sick at one time excrete too little, at another time too much; again from one part too little, at another time too much; and these classes of diseases are sometimes acute, sometimes chronic, at times on the increase, at times constant, at times diminishing. Once it has been recognized, then, which it is of these, if the body is constricted it has to be relaxed; if suffering from a flux, that has to be controlled; if a mixed lesion, the more severe malady must be countered first. Moreover, there must be treatment of one kind for acute diseases, another kind for chronic ones, another for increasing, stationary, or for those already tending to recovery. They hold that Medicine consists of such observations; which they define as a sort of way, which they name *methodos*, and maintain that medicine should examine what diseases have in common.[15]

We have here a precise formulation of the methodist doctrine at the approximate time of the formation of the sect. In essentials, this doctrine did not change, although the methodists were not in complete agreement about details. Unfortu-

15 Adapted from W. G. Spencer's translation of Celsus, Prooemium, 54 ff., vol. 1, p. 31.

nately, the writings of methodists other than Soranus are lost and it is to his works that we must turn for a study of details, always keeping in mind that Soranus does not represent the sect in all particulars. The fact that Galen, an enemy of the sect and a vehement critic of the methodists in general and of Thessalus in particular, does not attack Soranus, is suggestive of the differences in the sect, as well as of the esteem in which Soranus was held even by his opponents.

It has often been remarked that the methodist sect, because of its practical orientation and disdain of complicated theories, appealed to the temper of the Roman people.[16] However this may be, the fact remains that the sect was to play a greater part in the Latin West than in the Greek East. In the eastern parts of the Roman Empire, where Greek predominated, methodism apparently never took a strong hold. From the fourth century on we see a rising preponderance of Galen's authority in Alexandria, and by the early sixth century Galen's system of medicine had achieved the dominating position which it was to retain among the Arabic medical authors. Except as a gynecological author, Soranus did not play an important part in Eastern medicine; but the situation was different in the Latin West. Methodist influence remained strong among such early medieval authors as Vindicianus (fourth century) and Theodorus Priscianus (about 500 A.D.), and the influence and fame of Soranus equalled that of Galen. Not only were some of Soranus' works translated or abbreviated into Latin, but spurious writings, like the "Quaestiones medicinales" and "De pulsibus," appeared under his name. Only with the spread of Arabic influence, from the eleventh century on, did Soranus definitely move into the background

[16] See e.g. Theodor Meyer, *Theodorus Priscianus und die römische Medizin*, Jena, 1909, p. 9 f.

and Galen become the great unifying authority of scholastic medicine.

Soranus' Theoretical Concepts

The modern reader of Soranus' *Gynecology* will easily be provoked by his ambivalent attitude toward science. Soranus includes the physiological aspect in the disposition of the subject matter, but in the present work he restricts its discussion to the bare essentials, since, as he says, it is "useless for our purpose—although it enhances learning." [17] A similar statement occurs with regard to what is to be learned from dissection.[18] Possible causes of pathological conditions enumerated in the course of the book are frequently dismissed as irrelevant. All this is easily understandable as an expression of the general attitude of the methodist sect towards etiological research. However, the disdain which Soranus shows for what we may call science is more than compensated for by his learning. His interest expresses itself in various ways. Though he excluded a lengthy discussion of fertilization and embryology from the gynecological work, he wrote a special treatise on the subject.[19] To escape the blame of ignorance, he gave a description of the female generative organs [20] which was good enough to be included, more than 200 years later, in Oribasius' medical encyclopedia. He records the opinions of various medical authors, mentioning not only their names but very often

[17] Book I, 2; below, p. 4.

[18] Book I, 5; below, p. 7.

[19] In the *Gynecology* he refers to books "On the Seed" and "On Generation," probably parts of one work; see Kind, *loc. cit.*, col. 1126. From this lost treatise a doxographic excerpt has been preserved under the name of Vindicianus; see Werner Jaeger, *op. cit.*, p. 188 ff.

[20] Book I, ch. III.

the books from which he quotes. The "doxographic" parts of his writings were used by Greek and Latin authors and form an invaluable source for our knowledge of ancient medicine.[21] Finally, Soranus' scholarship manifests itself in his predilection for etymology. The manner in which he explains anatomical and medical terms may strike us as fanciful since it lacks all historical sense. Nevertheless, here too Soranus was considered an authority and used by later Greek etymologists.[22]

There is one field where the modern scientific reader will easily feel akin to Soranus, viz. the treatment of superstition. In his description of the ideal midwife, Soranus explicitly demands that she be free from superstition.[23] Where he takes occasion to relate popular or magical beliefs, we also find him on the side of the sceptic. We must not be misled by his references to the concept of "sympathy." As used by Soranus, this term merely means that physiological or pathological processes in one part of the body may lead to reactions in another part. The somewhat mysterious concept of a universal sympathy, favored by Stoics and Neoplatonists, seems to be foreign to him. When he assumes a "natural sympathy" between the uterus and the breasts [24] he tries to account for phenomena which we now ascribe to both hormonal and nervous influences. And when he attributes pathological disturbances and reactions to "sympathy," we must think of our own use of

21 See above, note 19. It is likely that Soranus was the source for the etiological sections in the so-called Anonymus Parisinus; cf. Owsei Temkin, Epilepsy in an Anonymous Greek Work on Acute and Chronic Diseases, *Bull. Hist. Med.*, 1926, vol. 4, pp. 137–44, where the pertinent literature is cited.

22 See Kind, *loc. cit.*

23 Book I, 4; below, p. 7.

24 Book I, 15; below, p. 14.

such terms as "sympathetic ophthalmia." On the other hand, Soranus has little use for action by "antipathy." There is one passage only [25] where he refers to such action without noting his dissent—and the genuineness of this passage was suspected by Ermerins, rightly, as I think.[26]

Nosology and Therapy

Soranus discusses diseases under the names and headings which were also used by other Greek physicians. He describes the clinical symptoms of each condition, possibly also the location of the lesion, and he pays more or less attention to etiology. But whether explicitly or by implication, the methodist distinction between *status laxus*, *status strictus*, and *status mixtus* is always present. Now according to methodist doctrine, the status is indicated by the symptoms as they develop in course of the disease. It is easy to understand that diseases marked by a flux [27] would be classified as belonging to the *status laxus*, where a styptic treatment is indicated; whereas hysterical suffocation with its accompanying convulsions would impress the physician as presenting the *status strictus*,[28] requiring a relaxing therapy. It is largely from the treatment of diseases as recommended by Soranus that the underlying nosologic notion becomes evident. Again and again the physician is advised to use relaxing remedies to treat an existing tension or constriction or, vice versa, to use styptic and constricting medicaments where parts are relaxed.

However, in spite of the methodists' appeal to the direct

[25] Book II, 49; below, p. 120.
[26] Cf. below, p. xlvii.
[27] For instance gonorrhea; cf. book III, 45.
[28] Book III, 28; below, p. 150.

evidence presented by a disease, one often wonders how Soranus could know that a part was constricted, dense, and compact, or loose, lax, etc. The main technical terms of the methodists for the communities of *status strictus* and *status laxus* were the Greek words *stegnon* (*stegnōsis*) and *rhoōdes* (*rhysis*) respectively. But Soranus also likes to speak of constriction, tension, condensation, etc. using such Greek words as *pyknos* (*pyknōsis*), *tasis*, *diatasis*, *esphigmenon*, etc. The semantic distinction between the proper methodist terms and these latter words is not clear, and one has the impression that Soranus often slips into an assumed knowledge of the physical condition of an organ. Here the historical development of the methodist sect from the teachings of Asclepiades may offer a possible explanation. Asclepiades' theory of disease as caused by conditions of atoms and pores had been reinterpreted by the methodists but it had not been altogether eliminated. For instance, Soranus says that the nipples of the wet nurse should be neither too compact nor too porous. Conceivably this might refer to the impression on palpation. But the sequence makes it clear that Soranus actually thinks of the condition of the ducts or pores.[29] Again, when Soranus refers to the "shaking" that the infant suffered during delivery,[30] it is hard to tell whether he has in mind the mere fact of the strenuous passage or an upheaval of the atomic balance. In his discussion of the weaning of the infant, Soranus makes reference to the pores which can hardly be understood as other than the hypothetical internal interstices of Asclepiades.[31] Elsewhere, he himself speaks about "invisible

[29] Book II, 19; below, p. 92.

[30] Book II, 11; below, p. 80.

[31] Book II, 46; below, p. 117. The existence of ducts (*poroi*) was assumed by others than atomists too, see H. D. P. Lee, p. xvii of his translation of Aristotle's *Meteorologica* (Loeb Classical Library), and *Anonymous Londinensis*,

ducts,"[32] and indulges in downright physiology when he allows the infant to cry occasionally because "it is a natural exercise to strengthen the breath and the respiratory organs, and by the tension of the dilated ducts the distribution of food is more readily effected."[33] It is against the ever-present background of an atomic theory that we can best understand the strongly mechanistic trend in Soranus' thinking, his references to the dangers of bruising and squeezing, his frequent recommendation of passive exercise, i.e. rocking in a chair or in a carriage,[34] and, finally, the excellence of his obstetrical technique. Where Soranus has to deal with obvious mechanical factors, as in dystocia, he is not at all averse to adapting his treatment to the causes.

The close connection between pathology and treatment is also noticeable in Soranus' attention to the whole course of the disease and its differentiation into stages. In sketching the attitude of the ideal midwife, Soranus says that "she will not change her methods when the symptoms change, but will give her advice in accordance with the course of the disease."[35] A disease may run from its onset with increasing severity to its height and then decline. It may be acute or chronic or marked by attacks and exacerbations on the one hand, remis-

---

ed. Jones, pp. 88–89 (and footnote 2); 112–13, 114–15, 136, 138, and 140. But the assumption that Soranus borrowed this notion from other than atomist sources would add to rather than detract from his lack of strict adherence to methodism.

[32] Book I, 35; below, p. 34 and notes 66, 67. Invisible ducts are also mentioned in Caelius Aurelianus, *Acute Dis.* II, 98, and *Chronic Dis.* V, 105.

[33] Book II, 39; below, p. 111.

[34] Plato, in the *Laws,* book VII; 789 B ff. sets great store by the salutary effects of rocking movements. It seems to have been favored among Asclepiades and his followers. Cf. above, p. xxvi and Celsus, II, 14 and 15 (and Spencer's footnote, vol. 1, p. 180).

[35] Book I, 4; below, p. 6.

sions and intervals on the other.[36] As a general rule, Soranus advises a bland treatment, especially during the *epitasis*, the initial stage or attack, when the symptoms develop with greatest violence. Very drastic measures, however, are employed during quiet intervals, and especially if the illness becomes chronic. It is now that he resorts to the famous "cyclic treatment," aimed at altering the entire makeup of the organism. This treatment consists of two main cycles:

1. The "restorative" treatment (the *cyclus resumptivus* of Caelius Aurelianus) [37] during which the patient's strength is built up for:
2. The "metasyncritic" treatment (*cyclus recorporativus*),[37] characterized by a carefully directed diet and drastic local treatment. The diet includes acrid and "pungent" substances, and the local treatment is of a surgical or pharmacological nature (e.g. cupping with or without previous scarification, metasyncritic drugs). In very obstinate cases, vomiting is provoked: the patient is given radishes and an infusion prepared with honey in wine or vinegar (possibly also an extract of *scilla*), and the vomiting is then effected by inserting the fingers (or a feather) into his mouth.

The patient was not necessarily led through the entire cyclic treatment; parts of it, especially metasyncritic drugs and other measures might be prescribed during quiet intervals.[38] But the time element is always considered. It is one of the

[36] See also Drabkin's introduction, p. xix, to his edition of Caelius Aurelianus, *On Acute Diseases* and *On Chronic Diseases*.

[37] *Ibid.*, p. xx.

[38] The cyclic treatment is described at length in Caelius Aurelianus, *Chronic Dis.* I, ch. 1, p. 453 ff., while in the *Gynecology* a relatively detailed account occurs in book III, 14–16.

main characteristics of the "methodic" treatment of disease after which the sect took its name, and it shows itself also in a predilection for three-day periods, the so-called *diatritos*.

While the methodists, including Soranus, emphasized their theoretical differences from other sects and stressed their therapeutic principles, they were much less exclusive in their choice of drugs. The materia medica, of Soranus at least, shows fargoing agreement with that of Dioscorides and Galen, who in many cases used the same drugs for identical or similar conditions. There are, of course, exceptions; but on the whole Soranus seems even to presuppose a general pharmacological knowledge on the part of his readers. True, he wrote special pharmacological and therapeutic treatises [39] to which he occasionally refers in the *Gynecology*,[40] but such references are scanty and one has the impression that Soranus expected his readers to rely on their own knowledge, or to look for instruction to some general works on materia medica. Nor is this altogether astounding, for the sects differed mainly in the dietetic treatment of internal diseases. Apart from this there existed a large body of pharmacological and surgical practices shared by most ancient physicians, who took what seemed good wherever they found it. Even Galen was not above acknowledging his debt to Soranus in this respect.[41]

Soranus' Gynecology

A. CONTENTS [42]

In the initial chapters of Book I, Soranus outlines the ar-

[39] See Kind in *Pauly-Wissowa,* col. 1128.

[40] See below, pp. 135, 152.

[41] See Kühn's index in vol. 20 of his edition of Galen's works, s.v. Soranus.

[42] See Ilberg, *Überlieferung,* and Kind in *Pauly-Wissowa.*

rangement of his *Gynecology*. The work is to be divided into two main parts: the first on the midwife; the second "on the things with which the midwife is faced," i.e. midwifery.

The first part actually consists of only two chapters (3 and 4), sketching the necessary qualifications of a midwife and setting up an ideal to which the midwife might aspire. This raises the question as to what readers Soranus addressed in his *Gynecology*. Was it addressed to midwives, physicians, or a more general lay public? The domain of the ancient midwife extended beyond the field of obstetrics; it certainly included gynecology.[43] Soranus' first requirement of a midwife is literacy.[44] It would, therefore, be reasonable to assume that in his *Gynecology* he wished to present a comprehensive textbook from which prospective as well as practicing midwives could learn everything concerning their profession. Although, in all likelihood, Soranus also wrote a shorter catechism for midwives in the form of questions and answers, he might at least have thought of the midwife as a possible reader for the longer *Gynecology* too. Yet, to us it seems more natural to think of the latter work as having been addressed to physicians. There were at least some physicians who were called gynecologists, because they treated female illnesses.[45] Moreover, in complicated obstetrical cases, the male physician was called in,[46] and the number of medical authorities cited by Soranus indicates that the physician did not exclude obstetrics and gynecology from his field of knowledge. Soranus himself belonged to this category of physicians. He may even have been the most outstanding ancient gynecologist, and he certainly was the most influential author in the field for later

[43] Book III, 3.
[44] Book I, 3; below, p. 5.
[45] Book III, 3; below, p. 129.
[46] Book IV, 7; below, p. 184.

generations, although he did not deal with gynecology and obstetrics as exclusive specialties.

Today we are accustomed to draw a sharp line between medical works written for professionals and those written for laymen. We must beware of assuming that the same attitude existed in antiquity. The educated layman was much more likely to form his own judgment about medical matters, to criticize the expertness and skill of the physician he employed, and to treat himself or his family. In the case of Celsus, we even have a layman who compiled a classical medical text with such expertness that it is hard for us to believe that the author was not a medical practitioner.[47] In short then, the most likely answer to the question of Soranus' reading public would be that the *Gynecology* was intended for physicians, midwives, *and* laymen.

The second part of the *Gynecology*, comprising the bulk of the whole treatise deals with midwifery. Again we have a dichotomy: into things "according to nature" (*kata physin*); and things "contrary to nature" (*para physin*) or, in the terminology of our translation, "things normal" and "things abnormal." "Things normal" are dealt with in Books I and II. They comprise a short account of the female genitals (I, 6–18), the hygiene of female sexual functions and pregnancy (I, 19–65), normal labor and puerperium (II, 1–8), and, finally, infant care and children's diseases (II, 9–56). The diseases, although outside the "normal," are included so as to allow a uniform discussion. Thus the *Gynecology* of Soranus also presents an early pediatric text including its famous allusion to rickets.[48]

[47] See Temkin, *op. cit.*

[48] John Ruhräh, *Pediatrics of the Past,* New York, 1925, p. 4, rightly remarks that Soranus was writing on infant care rather than on infant diseases

Compared with modern knowledge, Soranus' ideas are rather uneven. In his anatomical descriptions, for instance, some parts are excellent; but the lack of a clear distinction between nerves and tendons is confusing, and his belief that the seminal ducts in women ended in the bladder,[49] as well as his denial of the existence of the hymen [50] is surprising. It is not altogether clear whether Soranus himself dissected and, if so, whether he ever had an opportunity to dissect a human cadaver. At the time of Galen, human dissection was no longer possible.[51] Soranus probably owed some of his anatomical knowledge to Herophilus who remained an authority on human anatomy even for Galen.[52] Regarding pregnancy, Soranus had but a scanty knowledge of its early phase, nor did he use the terms "embryo" and "fetus" in the modern sense, a difficulty reflected in the translation. The section on normal delivery is, unfortunately, fragmentary; here, more than anywhere else, we should like to possess the complete text.

Some sections are instructive because of the insight they give us into ancient practices, especially those connected with infant care. We learn about the ways of swaddling, bathing, massaging, and weaning children, the demands made on the wet nurse who, according to Soranus, "should be a Greek so that the infant nursed by her may become accustomed to the

---

per se. This fact explains why very common accidents only are mentioned and, on the other hand, diseases prevalent in older children omitted. For some discussion as to whether articles 43–45 of book II really refer to rickets, see George Frederic Still, *The History of Pediatrics,* Oxford University Press, 1931, p. 29.

49 Here he followed Herophilus; see below, p. 11.

50 Book I, 17.

51 See Ludwig Edelstein, The Development of Greek Anatomy. *Bull. Hist. Med.* 1935, vol. 3, pp. 235–48.

52 See Barbour (1914), p. 282 f.

best speech."[53] The discussion on how to recognize children worth rearing[54] suggests that children not considered worth while were somehow disposed of. This pagan practice stands in contrast to the medical ethics of the section on abortifacients and contraceptives. Here the physicians of Soranus' time were apparently divided into two factions of which one, citing the Hippocratic oath, rejected all artificial abortion because medicine should "guard and preserve what has been engendered by nature,"[55] while others admitted a medical indication for abortion. Soranus belongs to the latter group, but prefers contraception, as safer, to the destruction of the embryo. He emphatically demands of the ideal midwife that "she must not be greedy for money, lest she give an abortive wickedly for payment,"[56] a warning that would hardly have been necessary unless the temptation had been great in ancient Rome.

The remaining two Books deal with "things abnormal"; diseases treated dietetically find their place in Book III, whereas Book IV discusses conditions cured by surgery and drugs.[57] The distinction between dietetics, surgery, and pharmacology is an old one; Celsus states that medicine split into these three fields after the time of Hippocrates.[58] On the other hand, the distinction was not radical, especially concerning the relation of dietetics to pharmacology. Dietetic treatment,

[53] Book II, 19; below, p. 94 Soranus' preference for Greek women becomes quite outspoken in his allusion to rickets in Rome (book II, 44; below, p. 116, although Plato (*Laws,* book VII; 789 E) indicates that rickets was known in Greece too.

[54] Book II, 10.

[55] Book I, 60; below, p. 63.

[56] Book I, 4; below, p. 7.

[57] This disposition is outlined in book I, 2.

[58] Celsus, Prooemium, 9.

in the sense of ancient medicine, meant the prescription of a regimen in which not only food and drink, but rest, exercise and bathing, as well as drugs, found their place. Only where drugs alone were prescribed, or played the dominant rôle as in many surface lesions, was the treatment considered "pharmacological" in the strict sense.

To the modern taste, Book III is probably the least interesting of the whole *Gynecology*. It begins with a scholastic discussion of the existence of proper gynecological afflictions and it comprises several complaints which it is hard to fit into a diagnostic scheme. The pathology, in most cases, is utterly antiquated and so, of course, is the treatment. This does not exclude the possibility that many of the measures advocated were effective. However, modern therapy has developed in such a different direction, that few physicians will be able to claim experience with the methods advised by Soranus.

It is otherwise with Book IV, or at least with the few chapters preserved which deal with dystocia, retained secundines, and prolapse of the uterus. If Soranus' fame as an obstetrician has survived into our own days, this is mainly due to the obstetrical sections of his book. It must, of course, be realized that Soranus was much dependent on his predecessors, especially Herophilus and his school. Their works being lost, Soranus, apart from a short chapter in Celsus,[59] thus emerges as our main authority after Hippocrates. His *Gynecology* represents the body of knowledge gathered by the early second century A.D., sifted as well as enlarged by Soranus, but not altogether his original creation. This is quite evident in Soranus' discussion of the causes of dystocia where he accepts, in substance, the outline of Demetrius the Herophil-

[59] *Ibid.*, VII, 29.

ean,[60] limiting his criticism to the teleological tendencies of this "dogmatist." [61]

Demetrius divided the causes of dystocia into (a) those affecting the mind or body of the parturient, (b) those stemming from the fetus, or (c) those due to conditions of the birth canal.[62] Although there are some hints at skeletal abnormalities,[63] they are vague, and receive less attention than the condition of the soft tissues, psychologic factors, general or local disease, and the size, number, and position of the fetus. With regard to the latter, Demetrius, and Soranus too, distinguish three main groups: [64]

1. Longitudinal position. Head presentation with arms along the legs is considered the only "normal" position as it had been since Hippocrates.[65] Deviations of the head from a straight line, and prolapse of the arms (with parted legs) are considered abnormal, and so are foot presentations.
2. Transverse position with the side, back or abdomen presenting.
3. "Doubled up" with the head and legs, abdomen, or hips (buttocks?) presenting. The latter possibility is considered the worst.

[60] Book IV, 2–5.

[61] Book IV, 5; below, p. 182.

[62] Book IV, 2; below, p. 178.

[63] See below, pp. 176, 179, 182, 184.

[64] See Johann Lachs, Die Gynäkologie des Soranus von Ephesus, *Sammlung klinischer Vorträge,* begr. von Richard von Volkmann, N.F., Nr. 335, Leipzig, 1902, p. 722. See book IV, 3, below, p. 179f. Ignorance of the attitude of the fetus may be responsible for some of the fantastic positions described, especially those included below under "Doubled up."

[65] See Fasbender, *Geschichte,* p. 15.

In the report of Demetrius' views mention is made of podalic version in transverse position.[66] But it is not quite clear whether this refers to a dead or living fetus, since, a few lines further below, Demetrius (or Soranus) speaks of possible disembowelment of a "doubled up" fetus and Celsus [67] knows podalic version only in connection with extraction of the dead fetus. A lacuna in the text unfortunately occurs at the decisive point where Soranus himself describes the management of the transverse position.[68] The later paraphrase by Caelius Aurelianus suggests that in oblique position Soranus turned the fetus upon the head or feet, while in transverse position he preferred cephalic version.[69]

It is, therefore, all the more remarkable that Aetius, in the sixth century A.D., describes podalic version in impacted head presentation (possibly of the dead fetus). "If the head of the fetus is impacted, one has to turn upon the feet and thus extract it. But if [the head] is firmly impacted and cannot be pushed back into the interior, one must insert the curved part of the hook into one eye or the mouth or the neck and extract." [70] Aetius did not invent this procedure; the chapter is marked as taken from Philumenus. This author is now believed to have flourished after Soranus and to have borrowed from the latter. Here then is a gap in our knowledge, possibly due to the bad condition in which Soranus' *Gynecology* has come down to us.

There is reason to assume that the *Gynecology* was illustrated. None of the original illustrations have been preserved, but some idea of their character can be obtained from the il-

66 Book IV, 3; below, p. 180.
67 Celsus, VII, 29.
68 Book IV, 8; below, p. 189.
69 *Ibid.,* footnote.
70 Skévos Zervòs, *Aetii sermo sextidecimus et ultimus,* Leipzig, 1901, p. 31.

lustrated copies of the Latin Muscio manuscripts, especially a Brussels manuscript of the IX–X century.[71] Crude as these later pictures are, they nevertheless yield an indication of what Soranus wished to clarify pictorially and we have, therefore, reproduced two of them in the present translation.

B. AFTERLIFE

Although Soranus was not a gynecologist in the sense of the modern specialist, his *Gynecology*, more than any other of his works, influenced medicine in the East as well as the West. We just mentioned Philumenus as an author dependent on Soranus, and we have to add, among late Greek compilers, Oribasius, Aetius of Amida, and Paul of Aegina. The sixteenth book of Aetius, in particular, rested to a very large extent upon Soranus who is used directly or through the medium of Philumenus. The influence of Soranus is likewise discernible in the gynecological sections of Paul of Aegina, although the relative brevity of his work led to many omissions. Yet it was Paul of Aegina, "al qawābilī," the obstetrician, as the Arabic physicians called him, who built the bridge between Greek and Arabic obstetrics and transmitted Soranus' teachings to the East.

Around 400 A.D. Theodorus Priscianus wrote his *Euporista*, the third book of which was based on Soranus' *Gynecology*. Originally composed in Greek, the work was translated, by the author himself, into Latin to make it popular in the West. Not much later, probably, the *Gynecology* of Soranus was paraphrased twice in Latin: first by Caelius Aurelianus, whom we have already mentioned as the translator of Soranus' *Acute* and *Chronic Diseases*. While a short fragment of these *Gynaecia* of Caelius Aurelianus had been known

[71] See Ilberg, *Überlieferung*, pp. 16 ff., and tables.

for some time, it is but recently that I. E. Drabkin identified this work within a gynecological treatise of a Latin manuscript of the thirteenth century.[72] In his edition Professor Drabkin shows that Caelius Aurelianus omitted most of the historical parts of the *Gynecology*, concentrating on the diagnostic and therapeutic parts which he gave in a version ranging from paraphrase to almost literal translation.

The other (and shorter) paraphrase stems from the pen of one Muscio (or Mustio), an otherwise unknown Latin writer of about 500 A.D. Muscio used the extensive *Gynecology* and, in particular, the shorter catechism which Soranus had written for midwives. The book was very popular during the Middle Ages, and together with its illustrations was used by Eucharius Rösslin in his *Der swangeren Frawen und Hebammen Rossgarten* (1513), which, in turn, was translated into Latin, French, English, Dutch, and Spanish.[73]

In Byzantine times, Muscio had also been translated into Greek. Since Soranus mentions a Greek author named Moschion,[74] the latter was wrongly believed to be identical with Muscio. Thus it finally came about that the Greek translation was retranslated into Latin by Dewez, as late as 1793. The latest critical edition of the Latin Muscio text was prepared by Valentin Rose in 1882.

C. MANUSCRIPTS, EDITORS, AND TRANSLATIONS

In spite of the great influence exerted by Soranus' *Gynecology*, the Greek text of the work barely survived in one badly

[72] I. E. Drabkin in *Isis,* 1948, vol. 39, no. 118, p. 238 f.

[73] See *Eucharius Rösslin's "Rosengarten"* . . . Begleit-Text von Gustav Klein, München, 1910 [Alte Meister der Medizin und Naturkunde, 2]. Rösslin's work and its connection with Muscio and Soranus have been discussed by E. Ingerslev in the *Journal of Obstetrics and Gynaecology of the British Empire,* Jan.–Feb., 1909.

[74] See below, p. 103.

corrupted manuscript, the Codex Parisinus Graecus 2153 of the Bibliothèque Nationale. This manuscript, written in the fifteenth century, comprises several medical writings. On leaves 218 to 284, it contains the index and text of a gynecological work without any author's name in the title. However, it was not difficult to see that this work was associated with Soranus. Some of its sections, transmitted in other Greek manuscripts under Soranus' name, gave a clear hint, and an unknown person had even entered the notation "this is Soranus." [75]

The discovery of the real significance of this gynecological work must be credited to the German physician-scholar Friedrich Reinhold Dietz. While in Paris in 1830–31, he copied the text and had begun publishing it, when he died in 1836. The work was brought out by a relative of Dietz, in 1838, under the title, *The Remains of Soranus the Ephesian's On Obstetrics and Women's Diseases*.[76] This title, however, was misleading. The gynecological treatise preserved in the Parisinus Graecus 2153 does not represent Soranus' work in its original form. It is a compilation made up of large parts of Soranus' *Gynecology* with chapters from Aetius of Amida. Dietz himself may have been aware of this fact although, at his time, Aetius' sixteenth book had not yet been published in Greek.[77] His literary heir, at any rate, was not very circumspect, and so this edition of 1838 contains a mixture of Soranus and Aetius.

The merit of having attempted a reconstitution of the Soranus text in its original form belongs to the Dutch physician

[75] Ilberg, *Überlieferung*, p. 3.

[76] *Sorani Ephesii de arte obstetricia morbisque mulierum quae supersunt.* Ex apographo Friderici Reinholdi Dietz nuper fato perfuncti primum edita. Regimontii Prussorum, 1838.

[77] Ilberg, *Überlieferung*, p. 4.

Frans Zacharias Ermerins. The task was not an easy one, for not only had all material alien to Soranus to be recognized as such and eliminated, but, in addition, the original sequence of chapters had also to be reconstructed. Ermerins chose a way which, in principle, was followed by later editors too. He studied Aetius (in the available Latin translation) and utilized the catechism of Muscio. Besides, he perceived that in the introductory chapters of his *Gynecology*, Soranus himself had mapped out the arrangement of the work. Ermerins' edition, with a Latin translation, appeared in 1869.[78] It represented a great advance beyond Dietz, but it also suffered from serious shortcomings. For one thing, the source material which Ermerins utilized was doubtful in many respects. He had not been able to check the reading of the Paris manuscript; he had to use Aetius in Latin translation and Muscio, on the other hand, he used in the Greek translation edited by Dewez in 1793.[79] For another thing, Ermerins was very arbitrary in his reconstruction. Many of his conjectures were excellent and have been accepted by later editors, but very often he excluded words and passages without sufficient justification.

Obviously, the text of Soranus needed the knowledge of experts. Whereas Dietz and Ermerins had been physicians, Rose and Ilberg, who came next, were classical philologists. Valentin Rose engaged in the preparation of a revised edition of Soranus' *Gynecology* because he recognized it as the true basis of the Latin Muscio, in whom he was mainly interested. Nevertheless, he approached the task thoroughly. He collated anew the Paris manuscript and definitely established its unique character, showing that the two manuscripts Bar-

[78] See "Bibliographical Abbreviations" under Ermerins.

[79] Ermerins, p. xxiii.

berinus I, 49 (in Rome), and Vossianus graecus 8°, 18 (Leiden), both of the sixteenth century, which contain parts of the Soranus text, represented mere copies of the Paris manuscript.[80] He also used Greek manuscripts of the sixteenth book of Aetius.

Rose's edition appeared in 1882. A renewed impetus in the study of the Greek text of Soranus' *Gynecology* was given by the monumental edition of the Corpus Medicorum Graecorum, planned in the present century by an international association of academies, under the leadership of the Berlin Akademie der Wissenschaften, and partly executed when World War II stopped the work—temporarily at least. The task of re-editing Soranus fell upon Johannes Ilberg who spent about nineteen years on it. As a preliminary undertaking, he analyzed all the available source material minutely and investigated the tradition by which the Soranus text has come down to us.[81] Then, in 1927, he published his edition of the Greek text of Soranus' *Gynecology* (together with the few other short Greek treatises of the same author) as volume IV of the Corpus Medicorum Graecorum. The full title of the volume is: *Sorani Gynaeciorum libri IV, De signis fracturarum, De fasciis, Vita Hippocratis secundum Soranum.* Edidit Ioannes Ilberg. Lipsiae et Berolini in aedibus B. G. Teubneri, 1927. Detailed and careful indices, prepared by Ernst Kind, accompany the book. The present translation is based on Ilberg's Greek text with deviation in but very few instances.

Apart from Ermerins' Latin translation, Soranus' *Gynecology* has been translated into German by H. Lüneburg, with comments by J. Ch. Huber (1894),[82] and into French by

80 See "Bibliographical Abbreviations" under Rose.
81 The results of this preliminary work were published in his *Überlieferung.*
82 See "Bibliographical Abbreviations" under Lüneburg.

Fr.-Jos. Herrgott together with the Muscio catechism (1895).[83] The English reader who wishes to obtain an approximate idea as to the contents of the chapters missing in the Greek text of the *Gynecology* (and hence in this translation too), may be referred to Francis Adams' translation of Paul of Aegina, and the recently published translation (from the Latin) of Aetius by James V. Ricci.[84]

83 *Soranus d'Éphèse, Traité des maladies des femmes, et Moschion, son abbréviateur et traducteur.* Traduits et annotés par le Dr. Fr.-Jos. Herrgott. Nancy, 1895.

84 *Aetios of Amida,* The Gynaecology and Obstetrics of the VIth Century, A.D. Translated from the Latin edition of Cornarius, 1542, and fully annotated by James V. Ricci. Philadelphia, The Blakiston Company, 1950.

SORANUS'
GYNECOLOGY

The Roman numerals denote chapters, and the Arabic numerals, articles. Numbers in brackets refer to the enumeration in Rose's edition which divided the whole *Gynecology* into two books only.

Following Ilberg's edition, angular brackets denote that the words within them are missing in the manuscript and were added by the editor.

In the transcription of Greek words, the letter upsilon has been rendered by "y" in order to elucidate the etymological relationship of such words as hysteria and hystera. However, where upsilon appears as part of a diphthong, it has been transcribed by "u." Names and places are given in their traditional forms.

‹ BOOK I ›

Into How Many and What Sections the Doctrine of Gynecology Ought to Be Divided.

1. Since the prefatory division of the subject-matter helps in elucidating the material, it is useful to begin the writing by dividing the subject into parts and sections. Now some people divide it into two parts: into theory and practice . . .[1] whereas practice, they say, is partly hygiene, partly therapy. And others divide it into a section on things normal and a section on things abnormal,[2] and still others divide it into physiology, pathology, and therapy.[3] We, however, divide

[1] The missing words may have been: "And further they divide theory into physiology, etiology and semeiology"; cf. Ilberg, p. 3, apparatus.

[2] Literally: "things according to nature and . . . things contrary to nature." This terminology implies that physiological conditions are in conformity with Nature whereas pathological conditions are contrary to her plans. It is this concept of Nature as the *norm* of life which justifies the more convenient translation by "normal" and "abnormal" adopted here and in many other places.

[3] This discussion of the division of gynecology reflects the various divisions of medicine current in antiquity; cf. O. Temkin, Studies on Late Alexandrian Medicine, *Bull. Hist. Med.* 1935, vol. 3, pp. 405–30. The Greek meaning of physiology, however, is broader than the modern one, extending into "natural philosophy."

the subject into two sections: into one on the midwife and into another on the things with which the midwife is faced.

2. More particularly we divide the section "on the midwife" into that on the prospective midwife (in which we inquire what persons are fit to become midwives) and into another on the person who has already become a midwife (in which we inquire who are the best midwives). Again, the section on the things with which the midwife is faced we divide into things normal and things abnormal. We divide the section on things normal into a chapter on the theoretical aspect of nature [4] (in which we consider seed and generation) and into a chapter on hygiene together with midwifery (in which we teach the care of the woman in pregnancy and childbirth, at the same time expounding the subject of the rearing of children). We subdivide the section on things abnormal into the part on the diseases which are treated by diet (in which we inquire further into the retention of the menstrual flux and difficult menstruation, hysterical suffocation and similar diseases) and into the part on diseases which are treated by surgery and pharmacology (in which we examine difficult labor, prolapse of the uterus, and the like).

Since, however, the theoretical part on nature is useless for our purpose—although it enhances learning—we have excluded it here, adhering for the present to the necessary matters only. First of all, we shall discuss the section on the midwife, then hygiene, and finally that on things abnormal. For the latter subject is more bulky and more difficult in its complexity and ought therefore to be imparted last.

[4] I.e. the part which, traditionally, belonged to "natural philosophy" and which Soranus rejected as useless for medicine (cf. below).

I. *What Persons Are Fit to Become Midwives?*

3. This paragraph is of use to prevent fruitless work and the teaching of unfit persons too accommodatingly. A suitable person will be literate, with her wits about her, possessed of a good memory, loving work, respectable and generally not unduly handicapped as regards her senses, sound of limb, robust, and, according to some people, endowed with long slim fingers and short nails at her fingertips. She must be literate in order to be able to comprehend the art through theory too; she must have her wits about her so that she may easily follow what is said and what is happening; she must have a good memory to retain the imparted instructions (for knowledge arises from memory of what has been grasped). She must love work in order to persevere through all vicissitudes (for a woman who wishes to acquire such vast knowledge needs manly patience). She must be respectable since people will have to trust their household and the secrets of their lives to her and because to women of bad character the semblance of medical instruction is a cover for evil scheming. She must not be handicapped as regards her senses since there are things which she must see, answers which she must hear when questioning, and objects which she must grasp by her sense of touch. She needs sound limbs so as not to be handicapped in the performances of her work and she must be robust, for she takes a double task upon herself during the hardship of her professional visits. Long and slim fingers and short nails are necessary to touch a deep lying inflammation without causing too much pain. This skill, however, can also be acquired through zealous endeavor and practice in her work.

II. *Who Are the Best Midwives?*

4. It is necessary to tell what makes the best midwives, so that on the one hand the best may recognize themselves, and on the other hand beginners may look upon them as models, and the public in time of need may know whom to summon. Now generally speaking we call a midwife faultless if she merely carries out her medical task; whereas we call her the best midwife if she goes further and in addition to her management of cases is well versed in theory. And more particularly, we call a person the best midwife if she is trained in all branches of therapy (for some cases must be treated by diet, others by surgery, while still others must be cured by drugs); if she is moreover able to prescribe hygienic regulations for her patients, to observe the general and the individual features of the case, and from this to find out what is expedient, not from the causes or from the repeated observations of what usually occurs or something of the kind.[5] Now to go into detail: she will not change her methods when the symptoms change, but will give her advice in accordance with the course of the disease; she will be unperturbed, unafraid in danger, able to state clearly the reasons for her measures, she will bring reassurance to her patients, and be sympathetic. And, it is not absolutely essential for her to have borne children, as some people contend, in order that she may sympathize with the mother, because of her experience with pain; for ⟨to have sympathy⟩ is ⟨not⟩ more characteristic of a person who has given birth to a child. She must be robust on

[5] Soranus rejects the dogmatists who base their therapy upon an inquiry into the causes of disease as well as the empiricists who mainly rely on observation.

account of her duties but not necessarily young as some people maintain, for sometimes young persons are weak whereas on the contrary older persons may be robust. She will be well disciplined and always sober, since it is uncertain when she may be summoned to those in danger. She will have a quiet disposition, for she will have to share many secrets of life. She must not be greedy for money, lest she give an abortive wickedly for payment; she will be free from superstition[6] so as not to overlook salutary measures on account of a dream or omen or some customary rite or vulgar superstition. She must also keep her hands soft, abstaining from such woolworking as may make them hard, and she must acquire softness by means of ointments if it is not present naturally. Such persons will be the best midwives.

5. Since we are now about to pass to the section on gynecological hygiene, it will first be necessary to explain the nature of the female parts. Some of this can be learned directly, some from dissection.[7] And since dissection, although useless, is nevertheless studied for the sake of profound learning, we shall also teach what has been discovered by it. For we shall easily be believed when we say that dissection is useless, if we are first found to be acquainted with it, and we shall not arouse the suspicion that we reject through ignorance something which is accepted as useful.

[6] Among the ancient physicians, Soranus is remarkably free from such superstitious beliefs as we find them even in Galen (see Introduction, p. xxxi).

[7] Soranus does not specify whether he refers to dissection of human cadavers or of animals only. His own criticism of dissecting as useless for medicine reflects the attitude of the methodist sect which rejected the scientific research of the dogmatists (see Introduction, p. xxx). On the whole subject of dissection in antiquity cf. L. Edelstein, The Development of Greek Anatomy, *Bull. Hist. Med.* 1935, vol. 3, pp. 235–48.

III. *What Is the Nature of the Uterus and of the Vagina?*

6. The uterus (*mētra*) is also termed *hystera* and *delphys*. It is termed *mētra*, because it is the mother [8] of all the embryos borne of it or because it makes mothers of those who possess it; or, according to some people, because it possesses a metre of time in regard to menstruation and childbirth. And it is termed *hystera* because afterwards [9] it yields up its products, or because it lies after [10] all the entrails, if not precisely, at least broadly speaking. And it is termed *delphys* because it is able to procreate brothers and sisters.[11]

7. The uterus is situated in the large space between the hips, between the bladder and the rectum, lying above the rectum and sometimes completely, sometimes partly, beneath the bladder, because of the variable size of the uterus.[12] For in children the uterus is smaller than the bladder (and lies, therefore, wholly beneath it). But in virgins in their prime of puberty, it is equal to the size of the superimposed bladder, whereas in women who are older and have already been deflowered and even more in ⟨those⟩ who have already been pregnant, it is so much bigger that in most cases it rests upon the end of the colon. This is even more the case in pregnancy (as can also be perceived by the eye) when the peritoneum

[8] This alludes to *mētēr*, the Greek word for mother.

[9] *Hysteron* in Greek.

[10] The Greek adjective *hysteros* (and its feminine *hystera*) has the meaning of "coming after," "following."

[11] Soranus (as Aristotle, "Hist. animal." III, 1; 510 b 13) tries to connect the name for the uterus with the Greek name for brothers *adelphoi* or sisters *adelphai*.

[12] For the understanding of this chapter, Barbour (1914) p. 273, footnote 1, points out that "this description is evidently taken from the dissection of a cadaver in the dorsal posture."

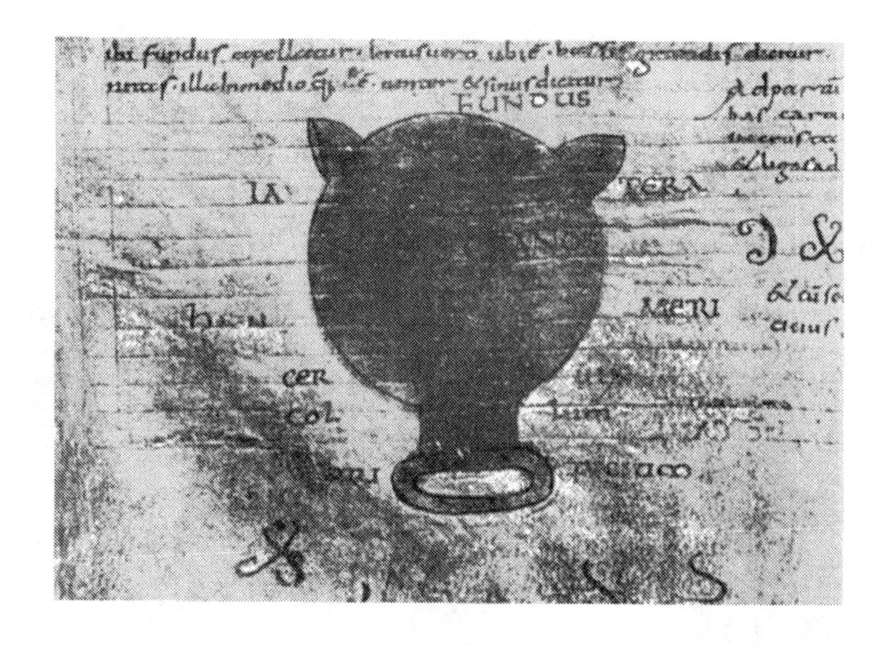

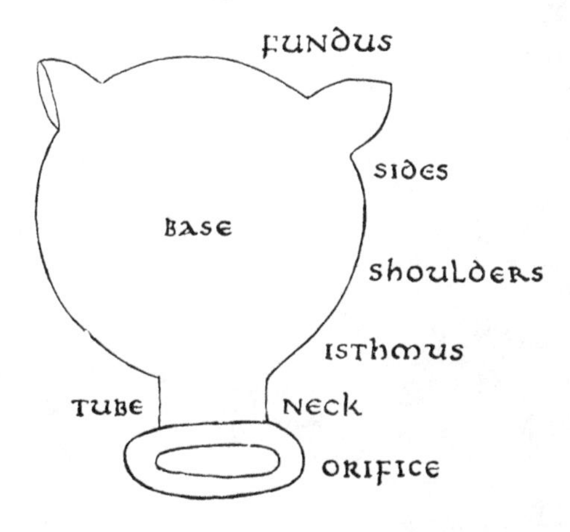

FIGURE 1

Above, picture of the uterus accompanying a Muscio text of about 900 A.D. *(Brussels MS. 3714; see Introduction, p. xliii). Below, same drawing with English terms used in Book* I, *9, of this translation.*

and abdomen are greatly distended by the magnitude of the fetus together with its membranes and fluids.

After delivery the uterus contracts, but its size is greater than it was before the pregnancy. Now the uterus is larger than the bladder, but it does not lie equally beneath it in all its extent. For anteriorly, the neck of the bladder (lying along the whole vagina and ending in the urethra) is more to the front and proceeds beyond the uterus. But posteriorly, the fundus of the uterus is higher than the fundus of the bladder and lies under the umbilicus. Thus the cavity of the bladder rests on the neck of the uterus, whereas its fundus rests on the cavity of the uterus.

8. By thin membranes the uterus is connected above with the bladder, below with the rectum, laterally and posteriorly with excrescences of the hips and the os sacrum. When these membranes are contracted by an inflammation, the uterus is drawn up and bent to the side, but when they are weakened and relaxed, the uterus prolapses. Although the uterus is not an animal (as it appeared to some people),[13] it is, nevertheless, similar in certain respects, having a sense of touch, so that it is contracted by cooling agents but relaxed by loosening ones.

[13] Notably Plato, cf. *Timaeus* 91 c, a passage on which Galen comments in "De locis affectis" vi, 5 (ed. Kühn, vol. 8, p. 425 ff.). Having quoted Plato, and having denied any wandering around of the uterus in the abdomen, Galen writes: "Yet somebody may ask us for the reason by which the uterus often appears drawn upwards and sidewards; for so do the midwives say . . ." And he answers: "For the tensions of the uterus are, I say, the causes why to the palpating midwives the cervix too appears drawn upwards and sidewards; for it is necessary that the cervix is drawn together with the uterus." The tensions of the uterus he ascribes to retention of the menses causing a plethora of the uterine vessels and ligaments. For a general discussion of Galenic gynecology and obstetrics, cf. Johann Lachs, *Die Gynaekologie des Galen,* Breslau, 1903 (Abhandlungen zur Geschichte der Medicin, IV).

9. The shape of the uterus:[14] it is not curved as in dumb animals, but similar to a cupping vessel.[15] For beginning with a rounded and broad end at the fundus, it is drawn together proportionally into a narrow orifice. The first and outermost part of the uterus has been called "orifice," the next part "neck," and the following part "isthmus," and the totality of these parts has been called "tube."[16] And after the narrowness of the "neck," the first parts of the uterus broadening on both sides are called "shoulders," the next "sides," and the remotest part "fundus." The underlying part is called the "base" and the whole space "cavity" or "hollow" or "sinus."

10. The orifice lies in the middle of the vagina, for the neck of the uterus is enclosed tightly by <the inner part of the vagina, while the outer part of the vagina ends in>[17] the labia. From the latter the orifice is more or less distant, according to the age (thus in most adult women the distance is 5 or 6 fingerbreadths). The orifice becomes more easily accessible with the number of deliveries since the neck of the uterus elongates. It varies in size too, but in the natural state the orifice is in most cases as large as the external end of the auditory canal. Yet at certain times it dilates, as in the desire of intercourse for the reception of the semen, and in the menses for the excretion of the blood, and in pregnancy in proportion to the growth of the embryo. In parturition it

[14] For a better understanding of the following description cf. fig. 1 which reproduces the picture of the uterus as given in a Latin Muscio text of the IX–X century together with a redrawing in which the English equivalents of Soranus' terms have been inserted.

[15] Literally: "medicinal gourd."

[16] The word also has the meaning of "penis," and a comparison with the male penis occurs in I, 16 and 33 (cf. below pp. 14, 31).

[17] Ilberg's text here has a lacuna which we have filled by Kalbfleisch's conjecture (cf. Ilberg, p. 8, apparatus).

dilates further, to an extreme degree till it even admits the hand of a grown-up person. In its natural state in virgins, the orifice is soft and fleshy, similar to the spongy texture of the lung or the softness of the tongue. But in women who have borne children it becomes more callous and, as Herophilus says, similar to the head of an octopus or to the larynx, and it has been made callous by the passage of secretions and children.

11. Pre-eminently, the whole uterus is a sinewy [18] structure. For it is composed not of nerves only, but also of veins, arteries, and flesh.[19] Of these, the nerves take their origin from the membrane of the spinal cord, whereas the arteries and veins originate from the vena cava which lies along the spinal column and from the thick artery.[20] For two veins branch off from the vena cava, and two arteries from the thick artery; and of these one vein and one artery lead to each kidney, then before growing into the kidneys, they become divided and with two branches they implant themselves in each kidney and with two other branches they twine around the uterus. Thus it comes about that four vessels implant themselves into the uterus, two arteries and two veins. And from these one vein and one artery grow into each didymus.[21]

12. Furthermore, the didymi are attached to the outside of the uterus, near its isthmus, one on each side. They are of

18 Literally: "nerve-like" (*neurōdēs*).

19 The Greek term *sarx* which we have translated by "flesh" refers to muscular rather than fat tissue.

20 I.e. the aorta.

21 I.e. ovary; but the term didymus (lit. "twin") does not imply any notion that the female seed consisted of ova. The ovaries were discovered by Herophilus who probably also discovered the tubes and believed them to end in the urinary bladder (Galen, "De semine" II, 1; ed. Kühn, vol. 4, p. 597). Here as in most anatomical details, Soranus followed Herophilus. Cf. Diepgen, p. 135 f. and Lesky, pp. 159–63.

loose texture, and like glands are covered by a particular membrane. Their shape is not longish as in the males; rather they are slightly flattened, rounded and a little broadened at the base. The seminal duct runs from the uterus through each didymus and extending along the sides of the uterus as far as the bladder, is implanted in its neck. Therefore, the female seed seems not to be drawn upon in generation since it is excreted externally, a subject on which we have discoursed in the work "On the Seed."[22] And some people say, as[23] . . . too contends, that a cremasteric muscle is implanted in each didymus. And we ourselves have investigated this with our own eyes in a woman suffering from an intestinal hernia. During the operation, the didymus prolapsed since the supporting and enclosing vessels had become loosened; and the cremaster was dislocated together with them.

13. The whole uterus is composed of two layers which are arranged crosswise, similarly to the strips of papyrus.[24] The outer layer is relatively sinewy,[25] smooth, hard, and white whereas the inner layer is fleshy, rough, soft, and reddish. The latter is interwoven throughout with vessels, which, however, are more numerous and noteworthy in the region of the fundus, since it is here that the seed adheres and since from here the menses are produced. Now these two layers are interconnected by flexible membranes and nerves and if these are often stretched, the uterus may prolapse, the sinewy[25] layer remaining in its place, whereas the inner layer prolapses by eversion.

[22] This work is lost.

[23] Here only the letters *chios* are preserved, probably the ending of a name which Soranus quoted.

[24] Writing material was prepared from the papyrus plant by putting two layers of thin strips crosswise upon each other.

[25] Literally: "nerve-like."

14. Furthermore, in women who have had no children, the uterus generally has furrows in the region of the fundus, in most cases two folded in like a cap. But in women who have given birth, the whole uterus stretches and becomes round. Diocles says that there are also what are called suckers,[26] tentacles, and antennae in the cavity of the uterus which are protuberances similar to breasts, broad at the base, but tapering at the end and situated on the two sides; providentially created by nature, in order that the embryo may acquire the habit of sucking the nipples of the breast. But these statements are proven wrong by dissection (for one finds no suckers) and the account of them which has been brought forward has no foundation in nature as has been shown in the commentaries "On Generation."

15. Now one must not suppose the uterus to be essential to life. For not only does it prolapse, but in some cases, as Themison has related, it is even cut away without bringing death. And they say that in Galatia,[27] the swine are fatter after the excision of the uterus. If the uterus is diseased, it influences the cardia of the stomach and the meninges by

[26] Literally: "cotyledons," a name which was applied to the suckers on the arm of the Cephalopods (cf. Aristotle, "Hist. animal." IV, 1; 523 b seq.). Diocles of Carystus was hardly the first to attribute "cotyledons" to the uterus, since they were also mentioned by Hippocrates ("Aphorisms" V, 45), Aristotle ("De gener. animal." II, 7; 745 b seq.), and others (cf. Wellmann, *Fragmente,* p. 129). In this connection it is interesting to note that Herophilus compared the external orifice of the uterus in multiparae to the head of an octopus (cf. book I, 10; above p. 11).

[27] According to Galen ("De semine" I, 15, ed. Kühn, vol. 4, p. 570), female pigs were castrated in the Asiatic provinces of the Roman empire as far as Cappadocia. This would include Galatia which was situated between the "province of Asia" and the "province of Cappadocia." Galen says that castrated sows "all become similar to the castrated [males], very well nourished and fat, and that their flesh is sweeter than that of other females just as that of castrated males is sweeter than that of other males." But Galen refers to excision of the ovaries rather than of the uterus.

sympathy. It also has a kind of natural sympathy with the breasts. Thus when the uterus becomes bigger in puberty, the breasts become enlarged with it. The uterus itself brings the seed to perfection, whereas the breasts prepare milk as food for the coming child; and menses occurring, the milk stops, whereas lactation occurring, menstruation appears no more. Similarly in women more advanced in years, when the uterus is contracted, the breasts too become in a way shrunken. The size of the breasts diminishes too when the embryo is damaged. So if in pregnant women, we see the breasts shriveling and contracting, we predict an approaching miscarriage.[28]

16. Such is the nature of the uterus. The vagina, on the other hand, is also called the female sinus. It is a sinewy [29] membrane, almost as round as the intestine, comparatively wide inside, comparatively narrow at the external end; and it is in the vagina that intercourse takes place. The inner part of the vagina grows around the neck of the uterus like the prepuce in males around the glans. But the outer part grows to the labia, the posterior part to the buttocks, the sides to the fleshy parts of the hips, and the anterior part to the neck of the bladder. For, as I said,[30] the neck of the bladder extends beyond the orifice of the uterus and running along the vagina from above, its end grows into the urinary duct. Thus it is evident that the vagina lies beneath the neck of the bladder but upon the anus, the sphincter, and the extreme end of the rectum. In length, however, as we have shown above,[31] it varies not only in relation to age or intercourse

[28] For definition of the term (*ektrōsis*) cf. book III, 47; below p. 170.
[29] Literally: "nerve-like."
[30] Cf. book I, 7; above, p. 8.
[31] Cf. book I, 10; above, p. 10.

(when the neck of the uterus, elongating like the male genital, occupies a certain part of the vagina), but also due to the fact that in some women the uterine neck naturally protrudes further, whereas in others it is exceedingly small. In most adult women, however, the length of the vagina is six fingerbreadths. In virgins the vagina is flattened and comparatively narrow, since it possesses furrows held together by vessels which take their origin from the uterus. And when the furrows are spread apart in defloration, these vessels burst and cause pain and the blood which is usually excreted follows.

17. For it is a mistake to assume that a thin membrane grows across the vagina, dividing it, and that this membrane causes pain when it bursts in defloration or if menstruation occurs too quickly. And it is equally wrong to believe that this membrane, when it remains in place and is formed into a solid structure, produces the disease called atresia. For first, this membrane is not found in dissection. Second, in virgins, the probe ought to meet with resistance (whereas the probe penetrates to the deepest point). Third, if this membrane, bursting in defloration, were the cause of pain, then in virgins before defloration excessive pain ought necessarily to follow upon the appearance of menstruation and no more in defloration. And again, if the membrane formed into a solid structure caused the disease of atresia, it ought to be found constantly at the same place, as we see each of the other parts always remaining in its proper place. Now, however, in patients with atresia the membrane dividing the canal is sometimes found in the accessible parts of the labia, sometimes in the middle of the vagina, and at other times in the middle of the uterine orifice.

18. Such then is the vagina. And those parts which lie outside of it and are visible are called "labia," situated as if they

were the lips of the vagina. They are thick and fleshy and they end posteriorly in the direction of the two thighs as if diverging from each other; whereas anteriorly they end in the so-called "nymph." [32] This latter is the origin of the two labia and by its nature it is a small piece of flesh almost like muscle; and it has been called "nymph" because this piece of flesh hides like a bride. And beneath the nymph another small piece of projecting flesh lies hidden which is the end of the neck of the bladder. It is called the "urethra" and its rough wrinkled interior is called the "lip." The bladder in women is different from that in men; for in men it is comparatively big, and has a curved neck, whereas in women it is smaller and has a straight neck.

The nature of the female parts has now been established; and since the function of the uterus is menstruation, conception, pregnancy [33] and, after its completion, parturition, we shall use the natural order and speak first about the menses.

IV. *On the Catharsis of the Menses.*

19. The menstrual flux, since it occurs monthly, is also called *katamēnion;* [34] and *epimēnion* as well because it becomes the food of the embryo, just as we call the food prepared for seafarers *epimēnia.*[35] It is also called *katharsis*, since, as some people say, excreting blood from the body like excessive

[32] I.e. the clitoris.

[33] This is one of the few places where Soranus distinguishes clearly between conception and pregnancy; cf. book I, 43, below p. 42.

[34] *Katamēnion* is the singular of *katamēnia.*

[35] The various connotations of *epimēnia* are associated with the literal meaning "monthly."

matter, it effects a purgation of the body. In most women the menstrual flux is pure blood, but in some cases it is a bloody fluid or again a kind of ichor as in dumb animals. But none of these is abnormal since it is excreted without difficulty. In its connotation, therefore, the menstrual flux is blood or an analogous fluid, excreted naturally at definite times, mostly through the uterus. Now the previous words are clear; except "mostly" which is added to "through the uterus," because sometimes menstruation also takes place from the vagina.

20. Menstruation, in most cases, first appears around the fourteenth year, at the time of puberty and swelling of the breasts. Beginning from little, the amount of secretion increases and after remaining the same for some time, it diminishes again and so it finally comes to an end, usually not earlier than forty, nor later than fifty years. Now again "usually" has been added, for in some women menstruation continues till sixty. As a matter of fact, the increase and the decrease do not occur with such precision as Diocles supposed when he said that menstruation continues till the age of sixty, that <at first it is little, then> attaining its maximum remains constant for some time to stop again <afterwards> by a proportional process of diminution. For this is not always so; it increases and decreases in an indefinite fashion, varying from case to case. The maximal menstrual flux is two cotyles.[36] And this again we say estimating the majority of cases.

21. Some women menstruate one day, others, two days, still others, even a week or more, but the majority, three or four days. This occurs monthly,[37] not with precision in all

[36] Approximately 15 ounces.

[37] In popular (and medical) usage the month meant a period of 30 days; cf. Pauly-Wissowa, XVI, 1, col. 46.

cases, but broadly speaking, for sometimes it is advanced or retarded a few days. For each woman it occurs at a stated time characteristic for her and it does not ⟨seize⟩ all women at the same ⟨period⟩ as Diocles ⟨said⟩,[38] nor, as Empedocles said, when the light of the moon is waning. For some women menstruate before the twentieth day of the month, others on the twentieth, and again some women menstruate when the light of the moon is waxing, some when it is waning and for the rest they menstruate on such days as is customary for them. Some people estimate the right measure of menstruation for all women from the summation of the days, for they judge that the natural excretion does not proceed beyond the third or fourth day. One ought, however, to censure these people, for some women naturally menstruate for a greater number of days, the same amount being distributed over many days; and on the other hand, more than the natural amount can be excreted in one day. One ought, therefore, to say that those women have menstruated in right measure who after the excretion are healthy, breathe freely, are not perturbed, and whose strength is not impaired, whereas all others have not menstruated in right measure. For the same amount of blood appears in both shortened and prolonged evacuations depending on age and the other circumstances, as well as on the fact that sometimes stoutening food, sometimes, however, pungent and attenuating food has been eaten.

22. But the amount of menstrual flow in women varies according to their nature as well as with age, season, physique, habits and mode of life and with certain other similar vari-

[38] The text here is uncertain. Caelius Aurelianus (*Gynaecia,* p. 8, 186 f.) has: "alie ante xx, alie, quod Diocles de omnibus estimavit, vigesimo admoventur die . . ." If Diocles referred to 20 days as the usual period this would explain Soranus' subsequent discussion of this period, although it may mean the last 10 days of the month.

ants. "According to their nature," because in some women more, in others less, menstrual blood is naturally excreted. "With age," for in women about to cease menstruating and in those just beginning, less blood is excreted. In such women, indeed, often only the area close to the uterus is moistened. For in very rare cases limited to women past puberty, a concentrated flow appears before defloration—however, as I said, it only stains the region.[39] "With the season," for in spring more blood is excreted, in summer less possibly, since then much evaporation takes place throughout the body; in autumn more blood is excreted in comparison to the summer, but less in comparison to the spring; and in winter, again, less than in autumn. "With the physique," for in very obese and stocky people the blood is lessened, perhaps because the material is spent on their good nutritional state. But in slimmer people with little flesh the blood is increased, for what nature does not use up for abundant nourishment, she adds to the excretion. "With habits and mode of life," ⟨for⟩ in women who lead an idle life the amount of blood is increased, whereas in those who lead an active life of whatever kind, it is less. And therefore, the amount decreases in teachers of singing and in those journeying away from home, especially in those going from an inland region to a place near the sea.

23. Sometimes it is also natural not to menstruate at all, not only during infancy or old age, but also in women engaged in singing contests, since the material[40] is forced to move around and is utterly consumed. It is natural too in persons

[39] The meaning seems to be that in the majority of these cases the excreted matter is thin, and even where it is more concentrated (in some women past puberty but before defloration) the quantity remains small. This interpretation is supported by Caelius Aurelianus (*Gynaecia*, p. 8, 192–95).

[40] I.e. the material from food which otherwise would have been elaborated into menstrual discharge.

whose bodies are of a masculine type, or when the material supplies the want arising from a long disease or when the blood is consumed on account of conception for the nutrition of the embryo. In some women, however, menstruation appears even after conception, either from the vagina or from the neck and sides of the uterus. For the attachment of the seed does not take place over the whole uterus, but in the fundus only. And sometimes a diapedesis of blood occurs from that part where the seed has not attached itself and therefore some women become pregnant again.[41] That it is at times natural for menstruation not to take place one should generally infer from the fact that no bad effects follow.

v. *What Are the Signs of Approaching Menstruation?*

24. One has to infer approaching menstruation from the fact that at the expected time of the period it becomes trying to move and there develops heaviness of the loins, sometimes pain as well, sluggishness, continual yawning, and tension of the limbs, sometimes also a flush of the cheeks which either remains or, having been dispersed, reappears after an interval; and in some cases approaching menstruation must be inferred from the fact that the stomach is prone to nausea and it lacks appetite. Menstruation which is about to occur

[41] The subject of "superfetation" was mentioned by Herodotus already who claimed (III, 108) that of all animals the hare alone could conceive during pregnancy. In the Hippocratic collection, a case history of alleged superfetation occurs in "Epidemics" v, 11 (ed. Littré, vol. 5, p. 210 ff.) while the theoretical side is stated in "On Regimen" I, 31 (ed. Littré, vol. 6, p. 506) and the first paragraph of "On Superfetation" (ed. Littré, vol. 8, p. 476). Aristotle discussed the subject at some length in "De gener. animal." IV, 5 and the "Hist. animal." VII, 4.

for the first time must be inferred from the same signs but above all from the growth of the breasts which, broadly, takes place around the fourteenth year, and from the heaviness, irritation and pubescence in the region of the lower abdomen[42] . . . it happens that women who have been forced to intercourse suffer this.

25. For the sake of proper care one should try from the thirteenth year on, before the menstrual flux is secreted, to assist the discharge to take place spontaneously and before defloration. For at the time of intercourse material is conveyed to the genitalia in females the same as in males, so that danger arises lest tension and inflammation be engendered if the organism has to make any effort towards the discharge. Therefore, her walk should be easy and deliberate, passive exercise[43] prolonged, gymnastics not forced, much fat applied in the massage, a bath taken daily and the mind[44] diverted in every possible way. For the body is relaxed together with the soul and bears the discharge without difficulty, unless the girl having been badly guided, is too pampered. For in that case one must tone up the body so that the uterus does not become softened together with the rest and therefore too weak for its proper function.

26. When menstruation first begins accompanied by the malaise which we indicated, rest is in most cases salutary. For just as people, full from a drunken bout, if they move vigorously may even lay themselves open to sickness, and as

[42] Ilberg thinks that the beginning of the following sentence is missing.

[43] "Passive exercise" means such exercise as swinging in a hammock or riding in a chariot whereby some rocking or shaking motion is imparted to the body without the patient actively exerting herself; cf. Introduction p. xxxiv.

[44] Literally: "soul."

those who have a congested head develop pain when they shout very loudly, in the same manner the uterus, filled with the menstrual material, through activity suffers compression accompanied by a feeling of weariness. And therefore one must make use of food which has wholesome juices and is adequate, and furthermore of vaginal suppositories of warm oil. But in women who have already menstruated often, each must be allowed to do according to her own custom. For some habitually take a rest, while others go on with moderate activities. But it is safer to rest and not to bathe especially on the first day. But in women who are about to menstruate no longer, their time for menstruation having passed, one must take care that the stoppage of the menses does not occur suddenly. For in regard to alteration, even if the body be changed for the better, all abruptness disturbs it through discomfort;[45] for that which is unaccustomed is not tolerated, but is like some unfamiliar malaise. The methods we employ at the approach of the first menstruation must now be marshalled forth during the time when menstruation is about to cease; for that which is able to evoke the as yet absent excretion is even more able to preserve for some time menstruation which is still present. In addition, vaginal suppositories capable of softening and injections which have the ⟨same⟩ effect should be employed, ⟨together⟩ with all the remedies capable of rendering hardened bodies soft. But if the menstruation is too much for the strength of the patient, or again, if it is impeded by abnormal factors, then there is need for therapeutic measures which we shall elaborate in the section on "things abnormal."[46]

[45] Literally: "suffering because of something strange" (*xenopatheia*); cf. below pp. 115, 118.

[46] Cf. book III, chs. I, XIII, and XIV.

VI. *Whether Catharsis of the Menses Fulfills a Helpful Purpose.*

27. Since one must aid those things which are helpful, but hinder those which are not helpful, we are compelled to discuss this subject. And one <must> point out two questions on the basis of the problem proposed: whether menstruation is helpful, first, with regard to health and second, with regard to childbearing, and the inquiry concerns both. Now, as Herophilus too recorded in his book "Against the Common Dogmas," some of our predecessors say that menstruation has a useful effect on health as well as on childbearing. Themison, however, and the majority of our people [47] find it useful only for childbearing, while some persons of distinction contend that it helps neither with regard to health nor with regard to childbearing. Herophilus and Mnaseas, however, say on the basis of different doctrines that in some women menstruation is profitable for health, in others, however, harmful. Now the first group [48] says that nature provides for mankind. She recognizes that men rid themselves of surplus matter through athletics, whereas women accumulate it in considerable quantity because of the domestic and sedentary life they lead, and mindful that they on their part do not fall into danger, she has provided to draw off the surplus through menstruation. Therefore, when menstruation is impeded, there follows heaviness of the head, dimness of vision, pain in the joints, sensitiveness at the base of the eyes, of the loins and the lower abdomen, discomfort, tossing about, upset stomach, and sometimes chills and fever;

[47] This refers to Soranus' own sect, that of the methodists.
[48] Those who believe menstruation good for health and childbearing.

and each of these difficulties is relieved when menstruation reappears.

28. In opposition to these people, one must say that the providence of nature has been disputed and that this proposition involves a decision which is more difficult than our problem: whether nature in her providence for men is able to measure their appetites so that they do not partake of too much food, or whether she can prevent the formation of surplus material. For if it is characteristic of nature to excrete providentially the excess, it would be in the power of the same nature to prevent the formation of excess material. But even if she created menstruation providentially, she did not contrive it for the preservation of health but for childbearing. Therefore, she did not bestow menstruation on those who are not yet able to conceive, like infants, nor on those who are no longer able to conceive, as is the case in women past their prime, but extinguished this activity upon the termination of its usefulness. And when menstruation is impeded, the body ⟨is⟩ trouble⟨d⟩ on account of that constriction [49] by which the menses are prevented from flowing. And therefore bringing on the menses has seemed useless since it does not remove the constriction or any of its symptoms, but when the constriction is dissipated menstruation reappears, as does the excretion of faeces and sweat. But sickness differs very much from health; and therefore that which is helpful in removing disease is no longer useful for the preservation of health. Thus venesection which dissipates the constriction does not preserve health.

But those who believe that menstruation does not even aid in childbearing say: menstruation occurs because the uterus

[49] This is a reference to the methodist concept of "status strictus," cf. Introduction, p. xxxii.

is ulcerated; but all ulceration is against nature and nothing which is contrary to nature is productive of natural activity, therefore menstruation is not useful for conception either. And further, some women conceive who have <not> menstruated at all, while others, conceiving before menstruation, have menstruated after conception. But one must censure these men too. For menstruation does not occur because the uterus is ulcerated, rather it occurs through diapedesis and profuse perspiration, in the same manner in which the gums too, when rubbed, emit blood without ulceration and as in fractures without wounds we find the bandages bathed in blood when the dressing is changed. And it is a mistake that some women conceive without ever menstruating. For if they are not cleansed by blood, they are at any rate cleansed by some other moisture, like some of the dumb animals. And after conception some women continue to menstruate as we showed before [50] from other parts and not from those to which the seed is attached.

29. Herophilus, however, says that on occasion and in certain women menstruation may be harmful, for some enjoy complete health while not menstruating, and often on the contrary when menstruating they become paler and thinner and acquire the beginnings of disease. Sometimes, on the other hand, menstruation may be advantageous in certain cases so that women formerly pale and meager, later on after menstruation have a good color and are well nourished. But Mnaseas says that some women are naturally strong, whereas others are naturally weak and among those naturally weak some are comparatively constricted, others comparatively lax.[51] And he says that in women whose nature is compar-

[50] Cf. book I, 23; above p. 20.
[51] Cf. Introduction, p. xxxii.

atively constricted, menstruation is salutary, whereas in those whose nature is comparatively lax, menstruation is not salutary, just as venesection, rendering the body more lax, is suitable for those suffering from constriction whereas it is harmful to those subject to flux, since it increases the already sufficient ease of passage.[52] But unaware he introduces ideas of Dionysius, calling "natural" a certain kind of constriction and laxity which is not healthy as has been pointed out in the second book of "On Communities."[53] Indeed, a natural state of relative constriction is still milder than the slightest condition of pathological constriction. Now venesection is harmful not only for those subject to flux, but also for those who suffer from a mild constriction, since it does more harm than good, the strength being called upon at the same time for restoration. In the same way menstruation may become harmful not only to those whose natural condition is comparatively lax, but also to those whose natural condition is comparatively constricted.[54] And both against him and Herophilus one must say that in regard to health menstruation is harmful for all, although it affects delicate persons more, whereas its harmfulness is entirely hidden in those who possess a resistant body. Now we observe that the majority of those not menstruating are rather robust, like mannish and sterile women. And the fact that they do not menstruate any more does not affect the health of women past

[52] I.e. ease of passage of particles through the ducts of the body.

[53] In his book "On Communities" Soranus apparently criticized Dionysius for defining conditions as natural which in reality were pathological, and he accuses Mnaseas of having fallen into the same error.

[54] The meaning seems to be that in slight pathological cases of constriction the disadvantage of bleeding (sapping the patient's strength) prevails over its benefit (release of constriction). Since constriction in the realm of the normal would be still milder than any pathological form, the loss of blood (menstruation) would have a very doubtful effect.

their prime, nay on the contrary, the drawing off of blood makes the majority more delicate. Besides, virgins not yet menstruating would necessarily be less healthy; if, on the other hand, they enjoy perfect health, menstruation, consequently, does not contribute to their health, but is useful for childbearing only; for conception does not take place without menstruation.

VII. *Whether Permanent Virginity Is Healthful.*

30. Some have pronounced permanent virginity healthful, others, however, not healthful. The former contend that the body is made ill by desire. Indeed, they say, we see the bodies of lovers pale, weak, and thin, while virginity because of inexperience with sexual pleasures is unacquainted with desire. Furthermore, all excretion of seed is harmful in females as in males. Virginity, therefore, is healthful, since it prevents the excretion of seed. Dumb animals also bear witness to what has been said; for of mares those not covered excel at running, and of sows those whose uteri have been cut out are bigger, better nourished, stronger, and firm like males. And this is evident in humans too: since men who remain chaste are stronger and bigger than the others and pass their lives in better health, correspondingly it follows that for women too virginity in general is healthful. For pregnancy and parturition exhaust the female body and make it waste greatly away, whereas virginity, safeguarding women from such injuries, may suitably be called healthful.

31. However, those of the opposite opinion contend that desire for sexual pleasures appertains not only to women but to virgins also. Some virgins, at any rate, they say, have

suffered more severe sexual passion than women; for the only abatement of the craving is found in the use of intercourse not in its avoidance. Maintenance of virginity, therefore, does not abolish desire. And as to the excretion of seed, some people say: Neither in males nor in females is it harmful in itself, but only in excess. <For> the body is harmed if the excretion is too frequent, but helped if it is spaced so as to get rid of the unwillingness to move and of discomfort. At any rate, many people after intercourse have been more agile and have carried themselves more nobly. Others, however, say that the emission of seed is injurious on the grounds that it brings about atony, and in this way sometimes actually harms people. But in another respect, namely for the unhindered discharge of the menses, occasional emission at the proper time, they say, is rather beneficial. For as movement of the whole body is wont to provoke sweating, whereas lack of motion holds it back and prevents it, and as the performance of the vocal function stimulates to an increased excretion the saliva which by nature accompanies the passage of the breath—in the same way, during intercourse the associated movement around the female genitals relaxes the whole body. And for this reason it also relaxes the uterus, so that menstruation is kept unhindered. Thus many women, menstruating with difficulty and pain because of a long widowhood, have menstruated freely after marrying again. Moreover, as to the pigs whose uteri have been cut out, they become stronger because they do not have the organ at all which has to suffer the menstrual excretion. Now just as a person cannot feel pain in the feet without having feet, nor would he have a squint if his eyes had been struck out, because he does not possess the member which would be diseased, neither is it possible for those who have no uterus to be affected by difficulties which originate in the uterus. But in virgins the uterus exists, so if they abstain permanently from intercourse, danger arises that the function of the uterus be destroyed too. And concerning the objection that women who have no intercourse escape the evil resulting from child-bearing, they say that by not having intercourse they are harmed in other respects much worse, the menstrual catharsis being hindered. Assuredly they become very fat and over-filled with complex substances when the matter which ought to be spent through menstruation is gradually accumulated. Permanent virginity, therefore, is harmful.

32. And such are the arguments of the two sides. We, however, contend that permanent virginity is healthful, because intercourse is harmful in itself as has been shown in more length in the book "On Hygiene."[55] Besides, even among dumb animals we see that those females are stronger which are prevented from having intercourse. And among women we see that those who, on account of regulations and service to the gods, have renounced intercourse and those who have been kept in virginity as ordained by law are less susceptible to disease.[56] If, on the other hand, they have menstrual difficulties and become fat and ill-proportioned this comes about because of idleness and inactivity of their bodies. For many of those who are thus kept virgins spend

[55] A Latin text edited by V. Rose (*Anecdota* II, p. 163 ff.) under the title of "Caeli Aureliani De salutaribus praeceptis" which probably is based on Soranus' work "On Hygiene" states (p. 201) that intercourse is necessary for conception but bad for the preservation of bodily health.

[56] Soranus probably includes the Vestals who had to guard the sacred fire. This would explain the reference to "observing and guarding" in the next but one sentence.

their time <observing> and guarding and do not participate in the necessary exercises, not even in passive exercise [57] and the benefit resulting from it, and, therefore, they are beset by the evils mentioned. Consequently permanent virginity is healthful, in males and females alike; nevertheless, intercourse seems consistent with the general principle of nature according to which both sexes, <for the sake> of continuity, <have to ensure> the succession of living beings. And this we must discuss next.

VIII. *Up to What Time Females Should Be Kept Virgins.*

33. Since the male merely discharges seed he does not run any risk from the first intercourse. Since the female on the other hand also receives seed and conceives it into the substance of the living being, and since in this respect one finds her endangered if led to defloration earlier or later than necessary, it is reasonable for us to inquire into the present problem.

Now some people have deemed it good for the female sex to remain in virginity so long as it has not yet an urge for copulation. For nature herself, in dumb animals and humans alike, has implanted certain torments and has set in motion appetites with regard to the proper time for intercourse, so that the body itself urges the approach to the pleasure of copulation. But it has escaped these people that dumb animals, directed by nature alone and blind necessity, of themselves contribute nothing to their desire. Therefore in most

[57] The translation of "passive exercise" rests on an emendation by Ermerins, the manuscript reading "winds" (*aerōn*). This original reading seems supported by the parallel passage in Caelius Aurelianus, *Gynaecia*, p. 12, 303.

of them the time of the appetite for copulation ⟨is fixed⟩ in advance, whereas in humans it is not fixed for a certain time, because often reason too stirs up the appetite for the sake of some novel pleasures or experiences. Now since virgins who have not been brought up wisely and lack education arouse in themselves premature desires, one must, therefore, not trust the appetites. It is good to preserve the state of virginity until menstruation begins by itself. For this will be a definite sign that the uterus is already able to fulfill its proper functions, one of which, as we have said before,[58] ⟨is⟩ also conception. ⟨For⟩ danger arises when the injected seed is conceived while the uterus is still small in size. The embryo, in consequence, is subject to pressure after its enlargement and will therefore either be entirely destroyed or lose its characteristics. Or, in any event, at the time of parturition it will endanger the gravida by passing through the parts around the orifice of the uterus which are still narrow and as yet imperfect. Thus it also happens that some embryos atrophy because the uterus has not yet been entwined with big vessels but only with small ones incapable of conducting sufficient blood to nourish the fetus. As a matter of fact in most instances the first appearance of menstruation takes place around the 14th year. This age then is really the natural one indicating the time for defloration. After a lapse of many years, on the other hand, defloration is not without danger either. For the neck of the uterus remains collapsed in the same manner as the genitals of men who have no sexual relations.[59] Thus the seed is formed and perfected into an organism in the roomy cavity of the uterus, but in parturition cannot easily pass through the narrow neck and brings about

[58] Cf. book I, 18; above p. 16.

[59] For this comparison cf. book I, 9; above p. 10.

great trouble and danger. Therefore the above-mentioned time at which the genital region has arrived at perfection and can endure conception is fitting for defloration.

IX. *How to Recognize Those Capable of Conception.*

34. Since women usually are married for the sake of children and succession, and not for mere enjoyment, and since it is utterly absurd to make inquiries about the excellence of their lineage and the abundance of their means but to leave unexamined whether they can conceive or not, and whether they are fit for childbearing or not, it is only right for us to give an account of the matter in question. One must judge the majority from the ages of 15 to 40 to be fit for conception, if they are not mannish, compact, and oversturdy, or too flabby and very moist. Since the uterus is similar to the whole <body>, it will, in these cases, either be unable, on account of its pronounced hardness, easily to accept the attachment of the seed <in the beginning>, or by reason of its extreme laxity and atony <let it fall again>. Furthermore they seem fit if their uteri are neither very moist or dry, nor too lax or constricted, and if they have their catharsis regularly, not through some moisture or ichors of various kinds, but through blood and of this neither too much nor, on the other hand, extremely little. Also those in whom the orifice of the uterus is comparatively far forward and lies in a straight line [60] (for an orifice deviated even in its natural state and lying farther back in the vagina, is less suited for the attraction and acceptance of the seed). Furthermore those who digest their food easily and have not loose bowels continually, who are of

[60] I.e. on an imaginary central axis.

a steady mind and cheerful (for chronic indigestion [61] is an obstacle to the fetus and a flux of the bowels allows what has been grasped to depart undeveloped; <the> sorrowful and passionate <state> of the soul, <on the other hand> expels the fetus <because of> the disturbance of the breath).

35. But some people have included those women who <show> neither joy nor sorrow in their expression while considering as less fitted those who quickly change color, especially if the color deepens.[62] For, they maintain, there is much heat in their desire causing the change and the darkening; by this heat the seed, dried up in some fashion, is destroyed. But it is a more reliable <and> fundamental indication <according to> Diocles, that women can conceive if in their loins and flanks they are fleshy, if they are rather broad, freckled, ruddy, and masculine-looking, whereas those with contrary characteristics are sterile, namely: the undernourished, the thin or the very fat, and those who are either too old or too young. But he pays the greatest attention to an indication by means of vaginal suppositories made of such substances as resin, rue, garlic, nosesmart, and coriander; for if upon insertion their property [63] is carried up as far as the mouth, he declares the women capable of conception; if not, the opposite is the case. And Euenor and Euryphon placing the women on a midwife's stool, made fumigations with the same substances.[64] All this is wrong. For a woman who was not fleshy in the loins, has conceived too, and the

[61] The manuscript here has a small lacuna, about eight letters wide.

[62] This follows Rose's text, p. 199, 18–20.

[63] I.e. their smell or taste.

[64] Antyllus, an approximate contemporary of Soranus, described fumigations for the treatment of hysterical suffocation and displacement of the uterus (Oribasius, *Collect. med.* 19, 2). The woman was placed upon the obstetrical chair and covered tightly with garments so that her face only remained free. Cf. also book III, 29.

substances made into suppositories and fumigations [65] will be carried up through certain invisible ducts [66] even ⟨if⟩ a person is unable to conceive. Asclepiades, in any event, says that if a cerate containing rue is applied to a patient with ulcerated legs, its distribution through the body will render him aware of its property.[67] As a general rule one must look for a woman whose whole body as well as her uterus is in a normal state. For just as no poor land brings seeds and plants to perfection, but through its own badness even destroys the virtues of the plants and seeds, so the female bodies which are in an abnormal state do not lay hold of the seed injected into them, but by their own badness compel the latter also to sicken or even to perish.

X. *What Is the Best Time for Fruitful Intercourse?*

36. Just as every season is not propitious for sowing extraneous [68] seed upon the land for the purpose of bringing forth fruit, so in humans too not every time is suitable for conception of the seed discharged during intercourse. Now so that the desired end may be attained through the well-timed practice of intercourse, it will be useful to state the proper time. The best time for fruitful intercourse is when menstruation is ending and abating, when urge and appetite for coitus are present, when the body is neither in want nor

[65] Literally: "what rolls."

[66] Literally: "ducts that may be seen by reason." Soranus here refers to the invisible ducts in the body, postulated by Asclepiades' atomistic theory. See Introduction, p. xxxiii.

[67] I.e. the patient will become aware of the taste of rue; see above notes 63 and 66.

[68] In contrast to humans where the woman also discharges seed from inside the body; see book I, 12.

too congested and heavy from drunkenness and indigestion, and after the body has been rubbed down and a little food been eaten and when a pleasant state exists in every respect. "When menstruation is ending and abating," for the time before menstruation is not suitable, the uterus already being overburdened and in an unresponsive state because of the ingress of material [69] and incapable of carrying on two motions contrary to each other, one for the excretion of material, the other for receiving. Just as the stomach when overburdened with some kind of material and turned by nausea is disposed to vomit what oppresses it and is averse to receiving food, so according to the same principle, the uterus, being congested at the time of menstruation, is well adapted for the evacuation of the blood which has flowed into it, but is unfitted for the reception and retention of the seed. And the time when menstruation starts is to be dismissed because of the general tension, as we have said; [70] likewise the time when menstruation is increasing and at its height because the seed becomes very moist and gushes forth together with the great quantity of excreted blood. Just as a wound does not unite if accompanied by a hemorrhage, and even if united temporarily opens again when the hemorrhage sets in, neither can the seed unite with and grow into the fundus of the uterus when it is repelled by the bloody substance excreted therefrom. Consequently, the only suitable time is at the waning of the menses, for the uterus has been lightened and warmth and moisture are imparted in right measure. For again, it is not possible for the seed to adhere unless the uterus has first been roughened and scraped <as it were> in its fundus. Now just as in sick people food taken during a remission and before the paroxysm <is

[69] I.e. the material to be discharged by menstruation.

[70] See above.

retained>, but is ejected by vomiting if taken during the paroxysm itself, in the same manner the seed too is safely retained if offered when the menses are abating. But if some women have conceived at another time, especially when menstruating a short while, one must not pay attention to the outcome in a few, but must point out the proper time as derived from scientific considerations.

37. We added "when the urge and appetite for intercourse are present." Just as without appetite it is impossible for the seed to be discharged by the male, in the same manner, without appetite it cannot be conceived by the female. And as food swallowed without appetite and with some aversion is not well received and fails in its subsequent digestion, neither can the seed be taken up or, if grasped, be carried through pregnancy, unless urge and appetite for intercourse have been present. For even if some women who were forced to have intercourse have conceived, one may say with reference to them that in any event the emotion of sexual appetite existed in them too, but was obscured by mental resolve. Similarly in women who mourn, appetite for food often exists but is obscured by grief from their misfortune. Indeed, later they are compelled to eat by reason of exceeding hunger, putting aside their resolve.

38. The time, therefore, is suitable which corresponds with the sexual desire, provided that the body is neither overloaded nor in want; for it is not enough to feel the urge towards intercourse unless the condition of the body is suitable too. We often crave food while the things already eaten are in a poorly digested and corrupted state, and if, at this time we partake of something, complying with the force of the appetite, we make this corrupt too. Similarly the proper time does not depend solely upon the craving for intercourse if in

addition we do not consider the rest of the circumstances; for in the more lecherous women the urge towards intercourse exists at any time. In fact, the body must be neither in want nor weak, for it stands to reason that together with the whole the parts too are weak. Thus if the uterus is too weak, it will be so, in all likelihood, regarding its functions too, and conception is a function of the uterus. Thus intercourse shall be practised neither when the body is in want, nor, on the other hand, when it is heavy as it is in indigestion and drunkenness. First, because the body in a natural state performs its proper functions but it is not in a natural state at the time of drunkenness and indigestion. And just as no other natural function can be effected in such a state, neither can conception. Second, because the seed when attached must be nourished, and takes food from the substance containing blood and pneuma which is brought to it. But in drunkenness and indigestion all vapor is spoilt and thus the pneuma too is rendered turbid. Therefore danger arises lest by reason of the bad material contributed the seed too change for the worse. Furthermore, <the> satiety due to heavy drinking hinders <the> attachment of the seed to the uterus. Just as in drunken people the wine, by vigorously rising up makes wounds difficult to unite, it stands to reason that the attachment of the seed is disturbed by the same cause.

39. What is one to say concerning the fact that various states of the soul also produce certain changes in the mould of the fetus?[71] For instance, some women, seeing monkeys

[71] The belief in the influence of the mother's impressions upon the fetus seems very old and widespread; cf. Fritz Kahn, *Das Versehen der Schwangeren in Volksglaube und Dichtung,* Diss. Berlin, Frankfurt a. M., 1912; and Max Wellmann, *Der Physiologos,* Leipzig, Dietrich, 1930, p. 42. Among the early Greek scientists, Empedocles is credited with the opinion that the embryo is shaped by the imagination of the mother during conception, and

during intercourse, have borne children resembling monkeys. The tyrant of the Cyprians who was misshapen, compelled his wife to look at beautiful statues during intercourse and became the father of well-shaped children; and horse-breeders, during covering, place noble horses in front of the mares. Thus, in order that the offspring may not be rendered misshapen, women must be sober during coitus because in drunkenness the soul becomes the victim of strange phantasies; this furthermore, because the offspring bears some resemblance to the mother as well,[72] not only in body but in soul. Therefore, it is good that the offspring be made to resemble the soul when it is stable and not deranged by drunkenness. Indeed, it is utterly absurd that the farmer takes care not to throw seed upon very moist and flooded land, and that on the other hand mankind assumes nature to achieve a good result in generation when seed is deposited in bodies which are very moist and inundated ⟨by⟩ satiety.

40. Together with these points it has already been stated [73] that the best time is after a rubdown has been given and a little food been eaten. The food will give the inner turbulence an impetus towards coitus, the urge for intercourse not being diverted by appetite for food; while the rubdown will make it possible to lay hold of the injected seed more readily. For just as the rubdown naturally aids the distribution of food, it helps also in the reception and retention of the seed, yester-

---

that frequently women had fallen in love with statues and images and had given birth to an offspring similar to these; cf. Diels, *Die Fragmente der Vorsokratiker,* 5. Aufl. 1. Bd. p. 300 (Empedocles A 81).

[72] I.e. not to the father only. According to Aristotle (*Politica* VII, 18; 1335 b), pregnant women should take a daily walk and nourishing food, but keep their minds quiet "for the offspring derive their natures from their mothers as plants do from the earth" (Aristotle, *Oxford transl.*). On ancient theories of heredity cf. Lesky.

[73] See book I, 38; above, p. 35.

day's superfluities, as one may say, being unloaded, and the body thoroughly cleansed and in a sound state for its natural processes. Consequently, as the farmer sows only after having first cleansed the soil and removed any foreign material, in the same manner we too advise that insemination for the production of man should follow after the body has first been given a rubdown. This does not contradict the statement in the book "On Hygiene" that the best time for intercourse is before the rubdown. For there the discussion was general, including the male sex, and concerned all possible intercourse; here, however, it deals exclusively with intercourse intended for childbearing. Healthful indeed as it is in itself to be given a rubdown after the disturbance arising from sexual pleasures, it is, on the other hand, equally advisable to keep quiet if the seed is to be retained.

41. But some of the ancients have also defined the proper periods as determined by external factors. Thus the time of the waxing moon has been considered propitious. For things on the earth are believed to be in sympathy with those up above; and just as most animals living in the sea are said to thrive with the waxing moon, but to pine away with the waning moon, and as in house mice the lobes of the liver are supposed to increase with the waxing moon but to decrease with the waning moon, the generative faculties in ourselves as well as in other animals are said to increase with the waxing moon but to decrease with the waning moon. Furthermore they say that spring is the supreme season for conception to take place. For in winter, bodies being condensed, seed is allegedly not easily conceived and even if conceived remains puny similar to the seed thrown upon the earth (for the latter too, in winter, is prevented from growing up, and of animals those born in winter are difficult to rear). Sum-

mer, on the other hand, because of the great evaporation makes everything weak, and therefore also the seed as well as the parts which conceive it, just as it weakens the whole body. But even without submitting the matter to reason, the evidence from phenomena is sufficient to put a bad face upon such things. For we see conception taking place in all seasons as well as being brought to a successful end. And if certain natures [74] unfitted to endure summer heat are worse off in summer or, on the other hand, those unfitted to endure winter cold are worse off in winter, we shall not pay attention to the seasons, but rather to the specific condition of the body. For as a general rule we premise a time in which the body is neither in want nor overburdened, but in every respect in a satisfactory state. And if at the changes of the moon some modification took place also in our bodies, we should in any event have observed it just as in mice and oysters. If, on the other hand, nothing of this kind has been observed to take place in our bodies, all such talk will be plausible but false.

XI. *Whether Conception* [75] *Is Healthful.*

42. Some people believe pregnancy to be healthful, because every natural act is useful, and pregnancy too is a natural action. Second, because some women, menstruating with difficulty and suffering uterine pressure, have been freed

[74] "Constitutions" would probably be a corresponding modern term.

[75] The Greek term *syllēpsis* connotes both conception and pregnancy. It literally means "laying hold of," "seizing." In the discussion of this and the following chapter, Soranus uses the term in its various meanings as it fits his purpose. The translation, therefore, also varies accordingly.

of their troubles after pregnancy.[76] Opposed to such arguments, one must say that menstruation too is a natural act, but not a healthful one, as we have recalled.[77] As a matter of fact if a thing is useful it is not in every case healthful as well. Indeed, both menstruation and pregnancy are useful for the propagation of men, but certainly not healthful for the child-bearer. For not by conceiving are they relieved of the preceding uterine troubles, rather, being relieved of the latter, they then conceive. Even granted that they are relieved by conception, conception is not a means of preserving health but an aid against disease; just as venesection does not become healthful because used as a treatment it resolves diseases. And according to what has been laid down previously, one has to point out that many inconveniences beset the pregnant woman who is heavily burdened and suffers from pica. Moreover, one must realize that the food sufficient for one organism has to be divided for the nourishment and growth of two organisms, so that it no longer remains sufficient for the gravida; for what is devoted to the fetus is of necessity taken away from the gravida. For it is not possible for her to take more food in proportion to the increase in consumption, since the process of digestion will not bear the management of more food. If, therefore, she takes as much food as she can digest and the part of the digested food offered to the fetus is taken away from the gravida, and if this diminution is not healthful, then conception is not healthful either. And that pregnancies bring about atrophy, atony, and premature old age, is manifest from the obvious facts and furthermore

[76] The author of the Hippocratic book "On Virgins' Diseases" (ed. Littré, vol. 8, p. 468) indeed urges marriage and pregnancy for virgins suffering from severe neurotic disturbances which he attributes to faulty menstruation.

[77] Cf. book I, 28; above p. 24 f.

from the similarity with the earth which latter becomes so exhausted from continuous production of fruit as not to be able to yield fruit every year.

XII. *What Are the Signs of Conception?*

43. Conception has been named from its being a retention of the seed, and it is called *kyēsis* on account of its being a *keuthēsis,* that is a concealment; for *keuthein* means to conceal and that which is conceived in the uterus is concealed. But as to connotation, conception is the prolonged hold on the seed or an embryo or embryos in the uterus from a natural cause. "Hold," because conception is a detention; and "prolonged," because sometimes the seed is laid hold of temporarily and is immediately ejected again, and this is not conception. "On the seed <or> an embryo," because during the first period, when the offspring is still unshapen, this is conception of the seed; but after the first period, when the fetus is already moulded and it is no longer seed, conception does not cease to be, although it is not pregnancy with seed, but with an embryo. For the seed has been changed and is already a nature, in process of time soul too, and no longer seed.[78] Therefore, some people, establishing a subdivision of conception, call the incomplete the first, and the complete the second. And in order to include the two forms, we said "on

[78] Galen (*On the Natural Faculties* II, 3; p. 131) writes: "For that which was previously semen, when it begins to procreate and to shape the animal, becomes, so to say, a special *nature.*" The translator, Dr. Brock, explains this last expression as meaning: "The spermatozoon now becomes an 'organism' proper." Soranus seems to think that in the process of development the embryo acquires an organismic status of its own and, finally, psychic individuality.

the seed or an embryo," and since sometimes also twins or triplets are conceived, we added "<or> embryos." "In the uterus," as prolonged detention of the seed in any part is not conception unless in the uterus; for while the seed is confined in the seminal ducts, it is detained for a long time, but this is not conception. Finally there is added: "from a natural cause," since often the seed is also retained, even for a long time and in the uterus, when the orifice of the uterus is closed by reason of coldness; or the fetus is retained in difficult labor. But such retention is not conception, for it is not brought about by the natural function, rather by one which is contrary to nature. There is also a difference between reception and conception. For reception is the conveying of the seed to the fundus of the uterus, whereas conception is its retention and attachment after its conveyance; furthermore reception refers to the seed only, while conception refers to the embryo too.

44. These points have thus been cleared up. Now one must realize that some people have said that <conception> cannot be recognized.[79] Yet in our opinion, one must work out the evidence for conception from the many signs lumped together and by their differentiation. For instance from the facts: that at the end of intercourse the woman has been conscious of a shivering sensation, that the orifice of the uterus is closed but soft to the touch and lacking in resistance (for in coldness and inflammation it closes too, but there is roughness and hardness),[80] that the vagina is not kept moist

[79] Caelius Aurelianus (*Gynaecia,* p. 18, 445 ff.) adds that in the opinion of some people conception is marked by an aversion to sexual intercourse. He denies it by pointing out that even among animals, hens and she-hares do not refuse intercourse after conception and that women too enjoy it "until the day of delivery."

[80] Cf. book II, 1; below p. 70.

by the seed or only slightly, the whole of the moisture <or> its greater part having been directed upward. Later on also from the facts: that the monthly catharsis is held back or appears only slightly, that the loins feel rather heavy, that imperceptibly the breasts swell, which is accompanied by a certain painful feeling, that the stomach is upset, that the vessels on the breast appear prominent and livid and the region below the eyes greenish, that sometimes darkish splotches spread over the region above the eyes and so-called freckles develop. And still later, from the appearance of the pica and from the swelling of the abdomen in proportion to the passage of time; and then from the fact that the gravida perceives the movement of the fetus.

XIII. *What Are the Signs, According to the Ancients, Whether the Fetus Is Male or Female?*

45. Hippocrates says [81] that <the signs> of pregnancy with a male are: the gravida has better color, moves with more ease, her right breast is bigger, firmer, fuller, and in particular the nipple is swollen. Whereas the signs with a female are that together with pallor, the left breast is more enlarged and in particular the nipple. This conclusion he has reached from a false assumption. For he believed a male to be formed if the seed were conceived in the right part of the uterus, a female, on the other hand, if in the left part.[82] But in the

[81] Signs indicating the sex of the fetus are mentioned in the following Hippocratic works: "Aphorisms" v, 42 (ed. Littré, vol. 4, p. 547), "On Barren Women" (ed. Littré, vol. 8, p. 416, no. 216) and "On Superfetation" (ed. Littré *ibid.* p. 486, no. 19). Soranus' account is more elaborate than the Hippocratic passages taken together.

[82] Cf. "Aphorisms" v, 48 (ed. Littré, vol. 4, p. 550) and "Epidemics" II, section 6 (ed. Littré, vol. 5, p. 137, no. 15).

physiological commentaries "On Generation" we proved this untrue. Other people say that if the fetus is male, the gravida will feel its movements to be more acute and vehement; if, however, it is female, the movements will be both slower and more sluggish, while the gravida too moves with less ease and has a stronger inclination to vomiting. For they say that the good color in women with a male child results from the exercise caused by the movement of the fetus; while the bad color in women with a female child is due to the inactivity of the fetus. But these things are more plausible than true, in as much as on the evidence we see that sometimes one thing, sometimes the opposite, has resulted.

XIV. *What Care Should Be Given Pregnant Women?*

46. The care of pregnant women has three stages. For the care during the first period is aimed at the preservation of the injected seed; during the second, at the alleviation of subsequent symptoms, such as the treatment of the pica which ensues; during the last period which is already close to parturition, it aims at the perfection of the embryo and a ready endurance of parturition. Of these, we shall at present make inquiry into the first.

When conception has taken place, one must beware of every excess and change both bodily and psychic. For the seed is evacuated through fright, sorrow, sudden joy and, generally, by severe mental upset; through vigorous exercise, forced detention of the breath, coughing, sneezing, blows, and falls, especially those on the hips; by lifting heavy weights, leaping, sitting on hard sedan chairs, by the administration of drugs, by the application of pungent substances and sternutatives; through want, indigestion, drunkenness, vomiting, diarrhea; by a flow of blood from the nose, from hemorrhoids or other places; through relaxation due to some heating agent, through marked fever, rigors, cramps and, in general, everything inducing a forcible movement by which a miscarriage [83] may be produced. Now of these things, those within our control ought to be eschewed, and one ought to keep the woman who has conceived quietly in bed for one or two days when she should use anointments in a simple fashion in order to strengthen her appetite as well as to aid the assimilation of the food offered her. But at the same time she should not allow massage of the abdomen lest through the associated movement in that region the attaching seed be torn off. One ought to anoint her with freshly extracted oil from unripe olives [84] and should give her less food and that of the cereal type. One ought to omit the bath, if possible, for seven days; for the bath, belonging to those things which loosen the texture of the whole body, will also help to enfeeble the delicate structure of the seed. Otherwise one would have to assume that wounds not yet safely united are further widened by a bath and the extremely compact bodies of athletes are relaxed, yet on the other hand, the seed will not melt away when its structure is still soft and has only just become solid. Hence there is nothing strange in the rejection of wine too for an equal number of days, so that the distribution of food may not become violent and overpowering. For just as the parts of broken bones, if not moved, become fused, so the seed too becomes implanted securely and firmly in the uterus, if not shaken by moving agents. On the other hand, to be sure, one must not continue this treatment for a longer

[83] For definition of the term "miscarriage" (*ektrōsis*) cf. book III, 47; below p. 170.

[84] See Materia Medica under "Olive."

period lest, the body becoming exhausted by the deprivation of wine and food, the uterus become languid together with it; rather one ought to change it little by little. As early as the second day, she ought to take passive exercise [85] in a stool or a large sedan chair (for being drawn by animals is to be rejected since it shakes violently); then she ought to take a short, easy walk in leisurely fashion lengthening it with every day; and she ought to partake of foods of neutral character, such as fish which are not greasy, meats which are not very fat, and vegetables which are not pungent. But she should avoid everything pungent, such as garlic, onions, leeks, preserved meat or fish, and very moist foods; [86] for the latter are apt to disintegrate, while pungent substances cause flatulence and besides are solvent and attenuating, and hence we approve of them in chronic patients for the removal of callosities for instance. But it is absolutely illogical not to realize that things which irritate, attenuate, and wear down the whole physique, and which dissolve callosities, that all these things, apportioned by distribution [87] to the various parts of the uterus, will soften the seed much more, which is like mucus as long as it is not yet held together by coagulation. And she must also beware of intercourse; for it too causes movement in the whole body in general and especially in the various parts about the uterus which need rest. For just as the stomach when quiet retains the food, but when shaken often ejects through vomiting what it has received, so also the uterus when not shaken holds fast the seed; when agitated, however, discharges it.

[85] Cf. above, p. 21.

[86] "Very moist" is a conjecture of Ilberg's. The Greek manuscript has "pungent" (*drimea*), whereas Caelius Aurelianus (*Gynaecia*, p. 20, 521 f.) has: "vel cibi nimium dulces."

[87] I.e. the process of distribution of food to all the parts of the organism.

She should take fairly warm baths for the sake of both the air and the water, without prolonged and copious sweating [88] lest the body become enfeebled and lose its tone. And the cold bath ought to be used in moderation too, so that no shivering sensation may arise. And after the rubdown she must fast until the body has become quiet and the disturbance of the breath and the agitation of the body fluids have calmed down. Later, for a fairly long period, she ought to drink water before meals or, if accustomed to it, a little weak wine.

47. Even if a woman transgresses some or all of the rules mentioned and yet miscarriage [89] of the fetus does not take place, let no one therefore assume that the fetus has not been injured at all. For it has been harmed: it is weakened, becomes retarded in growth, less well nourished, and, in general, more easily injured and susceptible to harmful agents; it becomes misshapen and of an ignoble soul. Can it be gainsaid that in the case of buildings, a house erected upon solid foundations remains indestructible for a long time, whereas buildings erected upon foundations that are not sound and solid fall down easily and at slight provocation? The construction of living beings is probably not different, except that they are underpinned, as it were, with different first elements and foundations.

If the seed is ejected,[90] the fact will be recognized from the extreme moisture of the vagina, but there will be corrective measures available against a repetition of the same mishap in conception. And to this end, if there is any bodily

[88] It has to be remembered that the bath in antiquity usually combined bathing in cold or warm water and perspiring in a heated room. On the whole subject cf. Oribasius, *Collect. med.* x, chs. 1–10, and the commentary of the editors, Bussemaker and Daremberg, vol. 2, p. 865 ff.

[89] Cf. above, p. 46.

[90] Cf. book I, 43; above, p. 42.

agitation, one must completely remove it; one must appease the soul, if the worries of life have troubled it; and if atony exists in the region of the uterus one must strengthen these parts together with the whole body. Such then is the care of the pregnant woman in the first period; and since with advancing pregnancy the so-called pica [91] arises, we also discuss it immediately hereafter.

XV. *On Pica (kissa).*

48. Some people say that pica (*kissa*) has been thus termed [92] metaphorically from a certain bird, the Kissa, for just as the winged Kissa [93] varies in its plumage and its voice, so the present condition is also productive of a varying appetite. Others, however, say that it has been termed this from the ivy (*kissos*), for it twines around in a way which also varies.

In most pregnant women it usually sets in around <the> 40th day, and then persists, generally, for about four months. In some women, however, it starts earlier or later and sometimes continues for a shorter, sometimes for a longer period, while in rare cases, it has been present until parturition but in others not at all. And those with this condition are affected with the following: a stomach which is upset, indeed full of

[91] See next chapter.

[92] We follow the reading proposed by Kind; cf. Ilberg, p. 35, apparatus.

[93] The Kissa is the Jay, *Garrulus Glandarius L.*, but the name included the magpie (*pica* in Lat.) as well (cf. D'Arcy Wentworth Thompson, *A Glossary of Greek Birds*, new edition, Oxford University Press, 1936, pp. 146–48). Soranus speaks of the winged Kissa possibly as distinguishing the bird from some fish, also called Kissa (cf. Liddell and Scott, s.v. 2). Through the Latin literature, "pica" has become more customary for designating the condition which Soranus terms *kissa*.

fluid; nausea and want of appetite sometimes for all, sometimes for certain foods; appetite for things not customary like earth, charcoal, tendrils of the vine, unripe and acid fruit; excessive flow of saliva, malaise, acid eructation, slowness of digestion, and a rapid decomposition of food. Some women are also affected with vomiting at intervals or at each meal,[94] or with a feeling of heaviness, dizziness, headache, discomfort together with an abundance of raw humors, pallor, the appearance of undernourishment, constipation; some also have gastric distention, or pain in the thorax, the same persons sometimes also show very slight fever and swelling up of the breasts (the swollen vessels are greenish in some, livid in others) and some display jaundice.

49. Now at the first sensation one must fast for one day so that the stomach, not being set in motion as is natural, may be kept undisturbed through rest. And one must not pay attention to the popular saying that it is necessary to provide food as for two organisms. For food which is not given to the body suitably decomposes and not only does not nourish but, in addition, harms the recently congealed seed just as it does the adult body. One must, therefore, fast. For travelers too, if they fast the day before, do not suffer from seasickness or not to such an extent. On the next day, one ought to give a rubdown with ointment, but should give little and easily digested food, like a soft boiled egg or a porridge, and some not very fat fowl, as well as water to drink, not much, but if customary cold, so that the abundance of fluids in the stomach may be checked.[95] On the following days, before

[94] This translation accepts Rose's text (see Ilberg, p. 35, apparatus) which seems supported by Caelius Aurelianus (*Gynaecia,* p. 23, 579): ". . . vomitus, nunc per intervalla, nunc iugiter perseverans."

[95] Cold water was believed a potent agent in causing or treating diseases of the stomach; cf. Celsus, I, 8.

anointing, one must first rub the body with pieces of soft linen to the point of moderate redness. After the first days the woman should take a comparatively hot bath, a little weak wine, and passive exercise, by means of movement in a litter and a sedan chair first, and then in a carriage drawn by animals. She also ought to promenade, exercise the voice and read aloud with modulations, take active exercise in the form of dancing, punching the leather bag, playing with a ball, and by means of massage. And in addition to bread she should eat any of those dry substances which are apt to strengthen the stomach. For thus the body is easily relieved from the evils of the pica, if at the same time the daily bath is relinquished and taken every second or even third day.

50. But if the stomach is greatly upset and full of fluids, one must apply over the stomach and the abdomen astringent embrocations made from the oil of freshly ground unripe olives, and in addition, bind about with wool; oil of roses, quinces, myrtle, mastich, spikenard also brace up the upset stomach. Or one may smear a cerate made with any of these substances over it. And if because of vomiting there is need of a more vigorous styptic action, one must use plasters, for instance dry dates soaked or boiled in tart wine or in diluted vinegar; apples or quinces boiled similarly, either alone or combined with the dates, or in addition to one of the cerates mentioned. If, however, we wish to increase the potency we may also add moist or dry alum, aloe, mastich, roses, saffron, bloom of the wild vine, pomegranate peel, *omphakion*, oak galls and hypocist or acacia, or the finest meal of barley. But if the vomiting and rejection of foods persist, it will be advisable to bind the extremities (for by their constriction the stomach is also affected) ⟨or⟩ to immerse them in hot water (for this too has a constrictive action on account of its

strength), and one must cause a wide-mouthed cupping vessel to adhere to the region of the cardia [96] by putting a rather big flame underneath, and if necessary, even a second one on the back, for they too restrain the flux [97] around the stomach in a similar fashion. And if the flux is combined with pain, one must apply a small poultice, styptic in action but nevertheless applied warm, for instance ground grain, especially barley meal or unsifted wheat, with diluted vinegar.

51. But above all one must take care to prescribe foods which are good for the stomach, easy to digest, and not readily decomposed, like soft boiled eggs, groats of spelt prepared with cold water, or with diluted vinegar, or together with the stones of pomegranate, or a very dry porridge of barley groats or best, one of rice. And of fowl those which are not very fat and have relatively dry flesh (such as francolin, ring-dove, partridge, wild duck, thrush, blackbird, pigeon, and domestic birds) and of these especially the breast. Of wild animals, the flesh of the hare or of the antelope, and of the others, kids, and the snout, feet, ears, stomach, and uterus of tender pigs. And of sea animals likewise those with firm flesh (for instance red mullet, crayfish, shrimps, trumpet-shells, certain varieties of oysters and mussels,[98] and purple fish). Of vegetables: raw as well as boiled endives, parsnips, purslane, plantain, wild asparagus. Of those from the store-room: olives pickled in brine, apples, quinces, and these preferably baked. For raw they are difficult to digest, boiled in water they lose much of their styptic effect, but well-crushed and sufficiently baked, besides keeping their quality they also gain digestibility. If, however, one wishes to have them boiled,

[96] Literally: "the mouth of the belly."

[97] Cf. below, p. 123.

[98] Soranus speaks of *sphondyloi* and *pelōrides* which probably were designations for certain kinds of oysters and mussels, but cannot be identified with any certainty.

they must be boiled resting upon rods or suspended by something, so that they do not touch the water but are boiled by the rising steam. One should also give pears or medlars or sorbs or a bunch of grapes conserved in an earthen pot or by hanging up (for fresh grapes cause flatulence), and almonds. But one must take care that none of the offered foods be dressed with a rich sauce; for a complicated and elaborate dressing causes slow digestion and decomposition of the foods.

52. But if, before taking food, some fluid has flowed in and lies on the surface of the stomach, one should not, short of actual stimulation, hinder its ejection by vomiting. For if not first evacuated, it becomes a cause of disintegration of the food introduced. But some of the heterodox [99] have even recommended, as an initial measure, first the drinking of lukewarm water, then inserting the fingers and bringing about vomiting. And the same people say that if an excessive amount of fluid is present, which is pungent and burning and therefore bites and inflames the stomach, one ought to give an infusion or a decoction of purslane to drink or purslane to eat and melon as well as cucumber seed together with water; one ought also to give sweet Cretan wine or southernwood or absinthium or an infusion of Syrian nard or Cretan goat's marjoram. If, however, there is a thick and viscous fluid, one ought to give radishes together with oxymel and preserved meat or fish, and the mustard remedy and hyssop boiled in hydromel. This is absolutely non-"methodic"; for one must not consider the variety of the humors, but the condition of the body. Furthermore, radishes are hard to digest, sweet wine causes flatulence, <and> absinthium is apt to produce miscarriage,[100] so that one must beware of giving these things.

53. One must oppose the desires of pregnant women for

[99] This refers to followers of sects other than the methodists.

[100] For definition of the term (*ektōsis*) cf. book III, 47; below, p. 170.

harmful things first by arguing that the damage from the things which satisfy the desires in an unreasonable way harms the fetus just as it harms the stomach; because the fetus obtains food which is neither clean nor suitable, but only such food as a body in bad condition can supply. For likewise, water streaming forth from the earth is transparent, if the earth is clean; if, however, it is muddy, the water is turbid. If, however, they feel wretched, though one should offer them none of these things during the first days, some days later one should do so; ⟨for⟩ if they do not obtain what they want, even the body, through the despondency of the soul, grows thinner. But that the harm may be the slighter, one must first point out to them that they should not partake of the desired thing before the rubdown of the body, when sometimes even the taking of that which is beneficial in kind causes harm. And they ought not to partake of it alone, but together with suitable food, ⟨in order that⟩ through the wholesomeness of the juices derived from the latter, it may be digested or at any rate, tempered. ⟨Moreover,⟩ one ought to give it in small portions, for the greater the portion the more the harm, and in between the other food, not before, or it will affect the bare stomach, nor later, for by lying on the surface it spoils the rest of the food too. Such, then, is the care of the pica, and in the following it is necessary to prescribe the care for the next period.

XVI. *What Is the Care from the Pica till Parturition?*

54. We have shown above, in what manner one must guide the gravida during the period of the pica, and this condition having been outlined, it remains in the following to describe

the care after the pica as well. Thus in proportion to her strength she must undertake various passive exercises,[101] promenades, vocal exercises, reading aloud, anointing, massage; she must partake of more plentiful food (provided she can handle what is offered), drink wine, indulge in the customary baths, and generally divert her mind,[102] and obtain sufficient sleep. When the body becomes more resistant, the gravida enjoys better health and is prepared to bear the pains of her travail with more strength, while the embryo partakes of more nutritious food which is healthful and sufficient.

55. At the seventh month she should give up the more violent movements and especially those caused by draught animals, while she should indulge in the others more cautiously. For being pulled about is dangerous in the beginning, when the seed is not yet strongly attached nor hardened into a coagulum and therefore easily suffers separation, and on the other hand later, ⟨because⟩ the perfected fetus is a heavy burden. At this time one must take care lest the chorion burst on account of too much tossing, and the fluid accumulated in it be evacuated and the fetus, drawn down in dry pregnancy, be endangered together with the gravida. (But during the mid-period the movement is free from risk, since the fetus is still of small size and safely attached, and the chorion is not yet greatly relaxed or distended, but rather gives support to the embryo.) In addition it is necessary to examine the abdominal enlargement and make sure that certain signs of imminent parturition, which we shall describe later,[103] are not present. For if some such sign is manifest, one must make

[101] Cf. above, p. 21.
[102] Literally: "soul."
[103] Cf. book II, 1.

preparations for parturition (for the evidence has shown that seven-months' children may also be capable of life) [104] —if not, one must practise what has been taught above. If, however, the breasts are considerably enlarged, one must take care, in rubbing, not to squeeze the tips, for being easily irritated, they are apt to develop an abscess; and for this reason women also slacken the customary breastbands to accommodate the enlarged parts.

56. With the beginning of the eighth month which people euphemistically call "easy," although it is burdensome and produces malaise and other distress, she must restrict still further the amount of food and must take exercise only in a litter or a big sedan chair, unless one desires to walk short of the point of exhaustion. And if the discomfort is greater, it will also be advisable to fast for one day so that the malaise can be dispelled by the respite. For one should not have recourse to the popular cold ablutions because the pregnant women cannot bear contractions [105] and if at the same time they are fed unseasonably, they suffer even greater harm. For if the food disintegrates, they are not only not nourished by the disintegrated things, but even burdened. And to some extent one must avoid the bath too. Sexual intercourse, however, is always harmful to pregnant women both on account of the tossing motion and because the uterus is forced to submit to a movement which is contrary to the process of pregnancy.

[104] The Hippocratic collection contains a special treatise "On Seven-Months' Children" whose author states that children of this age occasionally survive (cf. ed. Littré, vol. 7, p. 438). Aristotle ("Hist. animal." VII, 4; 584 b 3) affirms that seven months is the earliest age at which children can survive.

[105] This may mean that the cold water makes the organs (including the uterus) contract. Cold bathing had been among the favorite hygienic rules of Asclepiades (cf. Caelius Aurelianus, *Acute Dis.* I, 112). On the whole subject cf. the notes in Bussemaker-Daremberg's edition of Oribasius, vol. 2, p. 880 ff.

And even more so in the last months, lest because of it the chorion burst and the fluid which has been prepared for use in parturition be evacuated before the proper time.

If the bulk of the abdomen is hanging down under its weight, one must raise it by means of a broad linen bandage; one must place the middle under the bulk of the abdomen from beneath and carrying both ends up round the sides, one must cross them; then one must lay them over the back and shoulders and must fasten them down in front on the encircling band. One should also anoint the enlarged abdomen all over with a cerate containing oil made from unripe olives and myrtle, for if the skin is toned up it does not break, but is kept unwrinkled.[106]

After the eighth month, one should loosen the bandage since parturition is probably already imminent, and the weight will help towards a quicker delivery. The woman should indulge in baths more frequently in order to provide for relaxation of the parts and should swim in sweet warm water, for natural waters which have relatively pungent qualities differ in no way from drugs inserted for abortion. And more locally one must relax the parts by means of fomentations, sitz baths with decoctions of linseed or fenugreek or mallow, injections of sweet olive oil, and furthermore with vaginal suppositories of goose fat and marrow. And the midwife should herself dilate the orifice of the uterus, anointing it with her finger at frequent intervals.

106 This may conceivably refer to *striae gravidarum*.

XVII. *What Grows inside the Uterus of the Pregnant Woman?* [107]

57. Just as in eggs a membrane lies immediately beneath the shell and is closely attached to the surrounding hard crust, in the same manner, in pregnant women too, a membrane developed from the seed lies inside of the uterus. It is continuous in itself and has no orifices, it is grown to the fundus of the uterus from within and is composed of nerves, veins, arteries, and flesh. In color, it is of a purplish cast, in shape it is similar to the pouch of the Egyptian bean; [108] it is thick where grown to the fundus of the uterus, but membranous and thin at the other parts—for what reason, we shall say a little later.

This membrane has been called *chorion* and *angeion* and *deuteron* and *hysteron* and *prorrēgma*. *Chorion*, because it contains (*kechōrēkenai*) the embryo and the things belonging to it; or, as others say, because it consists of many units just like the choir (*choros*). *Angeion* (vessel), because it encases the embryo like a vessel. *Deuteron* (second) and *hysteron* (afterwards), because it follows after the removal of the fetus; and *prorrēgma*, because it is ruptured previously (*prorrēgnysthai*) and evacuates the enclosed fluid for a gentler delivery of the fetus.

Now from the more fleshy parts at the fundus a thin body descends and implants itself in the middle of the abdomen of

[107] In the Paris manuscript the order of the chapters is: XIX, XVIII, XVII, which Rose and Ilberg rearranged according to the sequence presented by Muscio. However, the original sequence is the one followed by Caelius Aurelianus, *Gynaecia*.

[108] Of the Egyptian bean (*Nelumbium speciosum*) Dioscorides (II, 106; vol. 1, p. 180, 12) says that its flower later on "bears a little bag similar to a wasp's nest in which there is a bean standing slightly out beyond the lid like a bubble."

the embryo at the place of the umbilicus (*omphalos*), and we call this very part which grows into the body of the embryo *omphalos*. It is composed of vessels, ⟨four⟩ [109] in number, two venous and two arterial ones, through which a sanguineous as well as a pneumatic substance is conveyed to the embryo for its nourishment. Empedocles believes that these vessels grow into the liver, Phaedrus, however, into the heart. But the majority believe that the veins grow into the liver, the arteries into the heart. Herophilus, on the other hand, thinks that the veins grow into the vena cava and ⟨the⟩ arteries into the thick artery [110] which extends along the vertebrae, but that before the implantation into the latter, they lie obliquely along the bladder on both sides. Eudemus, however, says that the vessels are simply brought together at the umbilicus of ⟨the⟩ embryo and that from here they part in the direction of the so-called horns below the diaphragm.[111] The fifth vessel, however, namely the "urinary," we designate in this way, whereas it is termed by the anatomists *ourachos* and this grows into the fundus of the bladder.[112] And through this the urine of the embryo is said to take its way into the chorion, while

[109] "Four" is a conjecture introduced by Ermerins, p. 94 of his edition. Actually Soranus counts 5 vessels, the fifth being the urachus (see below). Muscio I, 54 (ed. Rose, p. 19, 12) also writes that the umbilicus consists "of five things."

[110] I.e. the aorta.

[111] This may refer to the alleged "horns" of the uterus, which, according to some authors, extended from the uterus sidewise towards the iliac bones; cf. Galen, ed. Kühn, vol. 8, p. 889 f. where Eudemus is said to have called these parts "coils."

[112] This account contrasts with the following given by Galen ("De uteri dissectione liber," ch. 10; ed. Kühn, vol. 2, p. 907): "For the *omphalos* is nothing but the four vessels with the *ourachos* in their middle. The latter is the beginning of the allantoid membrane which, as we said, reaches the prominent parts of the fetus. It opens into the fundus of the bladder of the fetus by a wide and notable passage so that the bladder is connected with the allantoid membrane through the *ourachos* which lies between the two."

urination through the urethra takes place after parturition. For this reason, indeed, the membrane [113] is also thinner in the lower parts, because it is stretched and made thin by <the> pungency of the excess material [114] as well as by the large mass of the embryo. As a matter of fact, this excess material is useful first to float the embryo and, when the chorion bursts in parturition, to flow out first soaking the parts into slipperiness.

58. And so much for the chorion and the *omphalos.* But disagreement has arisen about the second cloak. For the majority say that in addition the embryo possesses another cloak, called the amniotic, which in dumb animals can be perceived since because of its toughness it does not become thin; whereas in humans, being worn thin by the pungency of the surrounding fluids, it is not found over the whole body, but only at such cavities as the nose, mouth and anus. And they say that it has been created by nature through necessity, so that the embryo may not be destroyed by drawing in the surrounding fluid which, consisting of excess material, is pungent and destructive. Some people, however, say that this membrane does not exist. For neither can it be found in parturition, nor would the whole membrane be useful, since the fluid is not so constituted; and even if it was so constituted, by habit it has become easy to recognize.[115] And besides, they say, it could not be drawn in through the mouth, since respiration takes place through the *omphalos;* influx occurs where something gives way, and since in embryos noth-

[113] I.e. the chorion.

[114] I.e. the urine.

[115] The meaning is not clear. The most likely interpretation is that if the fluid were pungent the fetus would have developed an instinctive reaction against it. Other possibilities are that a pungent fluid would easily be recognized by the usual effects, or by persons familiar with obstetrics.

ing gives way there could scarcely be an entrance for the fluids. And even if the embryo stood in need of a natural covering, it would be sufficient if the cavities alone were divided off by a membrane, without a cloak lying around the whole body; furthermore, since the mouth of the embryo as well as its anus is contracted, without their cavities being maintained, the assaulting substance is prevented from flowing in. But on the whole the fluid is not in the same cavity of the chorion as the embryo; rather it is in the thick mass of the chorion and makes a place for itself by infiltration, so that the chorion becomes twofold, and sometimes even threefold. For this reason, even though ⟨the⟩ engirdling layers often rupture and a moderate amount of fluid is discharged, still a continuous membrane meets the finger of the midwife; if, however, this membrane is torn asunder, with the evacuation of much fluid, the fetus also follows. In trying to evade this argument, the majority say that the fluids which appear beforehand are discharged because of an accumulation of hydatids: the hydatids burst, whereas the chorion remains continuous. We too agree with them, since above all the phenomena have testified to the structure of the amniotic membrane.

XVIII. *What Are the Signs of Impending Abortion?*

59. When abortion of the embryo is impending, a watery discharge appears in the aborting woman; then an ichorous one or a sanguineous fluid like the water in which meat has been washed. And when the moment for detachment has come, pure blood appears, and finally a clot of blood or ⟨some piece⟩ of flesh, unformed or formed depending on the different

periods. Besides, in most aborting women there is heaviness and pain of the loins, hips, and lower abdomen, of the groins, head, eyes, joints; a gnawing in the stomach, shivering and profuse perspiration, fainting, sometimes also a fever with chills, and in some cases hiccup or cramps or loss of voice. And these things mostly occur in women who abort from the use of a medicament. In those miscarrying without any interference, on the other hand, there comes first, according to Hippocrates, an unexpected shrinking of the breasts or,[116] as Diocles says, coldness of the thighs ⟨and⟩ a heaviness located in the loins around the very time of the delivery.

XIX. *Whether One Ought to Make Use of Abortives and Contraceptives and How?*[117]

60. A contraceptive differs from an abortive, for the first does not let conception take place, while the latter destroys what has been conceived. Let us, therefore, call the one "abortive" (*phthorion*) and the other "contraceptive" (*atokion*). And an "expulsive" (*ekbolion*) some people say is synonymous with an abortive; others, however, say that there is a difference because an expulsive does not mean drugs but shaking and leaping, . . .[118] For this reason they say that Hippocrates, although prohibiting abortives, yet in his book "On the Nature of the Child" employs leaping with

[116] Cf. Hippocrates "Aphorisms" v, 37 and 53, "Epidemics" II, 1, 6, and "On the Diseases of Women" I, 27.

[117] On the history of abortion in antiquity cf. L. Edelstein, *The Hippocratic Oath* (Baltimore, The Johns Hopkins Press, 1943).

[118] The Greek text at the end of the sentence is corrupt and Dietz' emendation, accepted by Ilberg, is not convincing.

the heels to the buttocks for the sake of expulsion.[119] But a controversy has arisen. For one party banishes abortives, citing the testimony of Hippocrates who says: "I will give to no one an abortive"; [120] moreover, because it is the specific task of medicine to guard and preserve what has been engendered by nature. The other party prescribes abortives, but with discrimination, that is, they do not prescribe them when a person wishes to destroy the embryo because of adultery or out of consideration for youthful beauty; but only to prevent subsequent danger in parturition if the uterus is small and not capable of accommodating the complete development, or if the uterus at its orifice has knobby swellings and fissures, or if some similar difficulty is involved. And they say the same about contraceptives as well, and we too agree with them. And since it is safer to prevent conception from taking place than to destroy the fetus, we shall now first discourse upon such prevention.

61. For if it is much more advantageous not to conceive than to destroy the embryo, one must consequently beware of having sexual intercourse at those periods which we said [121] were suitable for conception. And during the sexual act, at the critical moment of coitus when the man is about to discharge the seed, the woman must hold her breath and draw

[119] The Hippocratic Oath forbids the physician to give a woman "an abortive suppository." In the Hippocratic work "On the Nature of the Child," however, the physician advises a girl, believed to be in the sixth day of pregnancy, to expel the "seed" by leaping so that the heels touch the buttocks (the so-called Lacedaemonian leap). After the seventh leap the seed fell down with a noise (ed. Littré, vol. 7, p. 490). Some commentators apparently wanted to reconcile the contradictory views of the two Hippocratic writings by distinguishing between abortive remedies and expulsive measures.

[120] Soranus quotes the text of the Hippocratic Oath somewhat differently from the accepted literary tradition which reads: "I shall not give a woman an abortive suppository."

[121] Cf. book I, ch. X; above, p. 34.

herself away a little, so that the seed may not be hurled too deep into the cavity of the uterus. And getting up immediately and squatting down, she should induce sneezing and carefully wipe the vagina all round; she might even drink something cold. It also aids in preventing conception to smear the orifice of the uterus all over before with old olive oil or honey or cedar resin or juice of the balsam tree, alone or together with white lead; or with a moist cerate containing myrtle oil and white lead; or before the act with moist alum, or with galbanum together with wine; or to put a lock of fine wool into the orifice of the uterus; or, before sexual relations to use vaginal suppositories which have the power to contract and to condense. For such of these things [122] as are styptic, clogging, and cooling cause the orifice of the uterus to shut before the time of coitus and do not let the seed pass into its fundus. <Such, however, as are hot> and irritating, not only do not allow the seed of the man to remain in the cavity of the uterus, but draw forth as well another fluid from it.

62. And we shall make specific mention of some.

Pine bark, tanning sumach, equal quantities of each, rub with wine and apply in due measure before coitus after wool has been wrapped around; and after two or three hours she may remove it and have intercourse.[123]

Another: Of Cimolian [124] earth, root of panax, equal quantities, rub with water separately and together, and when sticky apply in like manner.

Or: Grind the inside of fresh pomegranate peel with water, and apply.[125]

[122] I.e. the drugs used as suppositories.

[123] The directions for the prescription are given in the second person, whereas the patient is referred to in the third person.

[124] Cimolus, one of the Cyclades in the Aegean Sea.

[125] I.e. as a vaginal suppository.

Or: Grind two parts of pomegranate peel and one part of oak galls, form small suppositories and insert after the cessation of menstruation.

Or: Moist alum, the inside of pomegranate rind, mix with water, and apply with wool.

Or: Of unripe oak galls, of the inside of pomegranate peel, of ginger, of each 2 drachms, mould it with wine to the size of vetch peas [126] and dry indoors and give before coitus, to be applied as a vaginal suppository.

Or: Grind the flesh of dried figs and apply together with natron.

Or: Apply pomegranate peel with an equal amount of gum and an equal amount of oil of roses.

Then one should always follow with a drink of honey water. But one should beware of things which are very pungent, because of the ulcerations arising from them. And we use all these things after the end of menstruation.

63. Moreover to some people it seems advisable: Once during the month to drink Cyrenaic balm to the amount of a chick-pea in two cyaths of water for the purpose of inducing menstruation. Or: Of panax balm and Cyrenaic balm and rue seed, of each two obols, <grind> and coat with wax and give to swallow; then follow with a drink of diluted wine or let it be drunk in diluted wine. <Or:> Of wallflower seed and myrtle, of each three obols, of myrrh a drachm, of white pepper two seeds; give to drink with wine for three days. Or: Of rocket seed one obol, of cow parsnip one-half obol; drink with oxymel.

However, these things not only prevent conception, but also

[126] The seed of the bitter vetch, *Vicia Ervilia,* often served as a measure of comparison; cf. Theophrastus, *Hist. plant.* VII, 6, 3; Dioscorides, IV, 150, 6; Alexander of Tralles 7, 4 (ed. Puschmann, vol. 2, p. 265).

destroy any already existing. In our opinion, moreover, the evil from these things is too great, since they damage and upset the stomach, and besides cause congestion of the head and induce sympathetic reactions. Others, however, have even made use of amulets which on grounds of antipathy they believe to have great effect; such are uteri of mules and the dirt in their ears and more things of this kind which according to the outcome reveal themselves as falsehoods.

64. Yet if conception has taken place, one must first, for 30 days, do the opposite of what we said earlier.[127] But in order that the embryo be separated, the woman should have <more violent exercise>, walking about energetically and being shaken by means of draught animals;[128] she should also leap energetically[129] and carry things which are heavy beyond her strength. She should use diuretic decoctions which also have the power to bring on menstruation, and empty and purge the abdomen with relatively pungent clysters; sometimes using warm and sweet olive oil as injections, sometimes anointing the whole body thoroughly therewith and rubbing it vigorously, especially around the pubes, the abdomen, and the loins, bathing daily in sweet water which is not too hot, lingering in the baths and drinking first a little wine and living on pungent food. If this is without effect, one must also treat locally by having her sit in a bath of a decoction of linseed, fenugreek, mallow, marsh mallow, and wormwood. She must also use poultices of the same substances and have injections of old oil, alone or together with rue juice or maybe with honey, or of iris oil, or of absinthium together with honey, or of panax balm or else of spelt together with rue and honey,

[127] Cf. book I, 46; above, p. 45.

[128] I.e. by riding in a carriage drawn by animals.

[129] Cf. above, p. 62 f.

or of Syrian unguent.[130] And if the situation remains the same she must no longer apply the common poultices, but those made of meal of lupines together with ox bile and absinthium, <and she must use> plasters of a similar kind.

65. For a woman who intends to have an abortion, it is necessary for two or even three days beforehand to take protracted baths, little food and to use softening vaginal suppositories; also to abstain from wine; then to be bled and a relatively great quantity taken away. For the dictum of Hippocrates in the "Aphorisms," even if not true in a case of constriction,[131] is yet true of a healthy woman: "A pregnant woman if bled, miscarries." [132] For just as sweat, urine or faeces are excreted if the parts containing these substances slacken very much, so the fetus falls out after the uterus dilates. Following the venesection one must shake her by means of draught animals (for now the shaking is more effective on the parts which previously have been relaxed) and one must use softening vaginal suppositories. But if a woman reacts unfavorably to venesection and is languid, one must first relax the parts by means of sitz baths, full baths, softening vaginal suppositories, by keeping her on water and limited food, and by means of aperients and the application of a softening clyster; afterwards one must apply an abortive vaginal suppository. Of the latter one should choose those which are not too pungent, that they may not cause too great a sympathetic reaction and heat. And of the more gentle ones there exist for instance: Of myrtle, wallflower seed, bitter

[130] The composition of this ointment that was imported from Syria seems to have been unknown to the physicians; cf. Galen, ed. Kühn, vol. 12, p. 543.

[131] Cf. above, p. 26.

[132] Hippocrates, "Aphorisms" v, 31. In the translation of Jones (Hippocrates IV, Loeb Classical Library, p. 167) this aphorism reads: "A woman with child, if bled, miscarries; the larger the embryo the greater the risk."

lupines equal quantities, by means of water, mould troches the size of a bean. Or: Of rue leaves 3 drachms, of myrtle 2 drachms and the same of sweet bay, mix with wine in the same way, and give her a drink. Another vaginal suppository which produces abortion with relatively little danger: Of wallflower, cardamom, brimstone, absinthium, myrrh, equal quantities, mould with water. And she who intends to apply these things should be bathed beforehand or made to relax by sitz baths; and if after some time she brings forth nothing, she should again be relaxed by sitz baths and for the second time a suppository should be applied. In addition, many different things have been mentioned by others; one must, however, beware of things that are too powerful and of separating the embryo by means of something sharp-edged, for danger arises that some of the adjacent parts be wounded. After the abortion one must treat as for inflammation.

⟨ BOOK II ⟩

1[xx]. *What Signs Precede Imminent Normal Parturition?*

1[66]. It is useful to learn the signs of imminent labor in order to prepare beforehand the things necessary for parturition. Around the seventh or the ninth or the tenth month in women who are about to give birth, there arise heaviness of the lower part of the abdomen and the epigastric region together with burning in the vagina, ⟨and⟩ pain in the groins, loins, and waist down into the region below the uterus. And the uterus advances further into the vagina so that the examining midwife can easily touch it, and its orifice expands and is also lacking in resistance, it stands open and is at the same time moist on the surface. In proportion to the imminence of parturition, the hips and the epigastric region fall in, while both ⟨the⟩ pubic region and the groins swell, and the desire to urinate becomes constant. A viscous fluid runs out, then in most cases blood too, when the thin vessels in the chorion rupture; while the finger inserted into the vagina meets with a rounded mass, closely resembling an egg. It has also happened that the distress was present because of an inflammation, but it will be distinguished by the fact that the orifice of the uterus is shut and dry.[1]

II[XXI]. *What Must One Prepare for Labor?*

2[67]. For normal labor one must prepare beforehand: olive oil, warm water, warm fomentations, soft sea sponges, pieces of wool, bandages, a pillow, things to smell, a midwife's stool or chair, two beds, and a proper room. Oil for injection and lubrication; warm water in order that the parts may be cleansed; warm fomentations for alleviation of the pains; sea sponges for sponging off; pieces of wool in order that the woman's parts be covered, bandages that the newborn may be swaddled; a pillow that the infant may be placed upon it below the parturient woman, till the afterbirth[2] has also been taken care of; and things to smell (such as pennyroyal, a clod of earth, barley groats, as well as an apple and a quince and, if the season permits, a lemon, a melon, and cucumber, ⟨and⟩ everything similar to these) to revive the laboring woman.

[1] Closure of the orifice (unless caused by disease) was generally recognized as a sign of pregnancy (cf. book I, 44; above, p. 43; Hippocrates, "Aphorisms" v, 51; and Galen, *On the Natural Faculties,* III, 3; p. 233). Herophilus, moreover, stated (cf. Galen, *ibid.*) "that up to the time of labour the os uteri will not admit so much as the tip of a probe, that it no longer opens to the slightest degree if pregnancy has begun—that, in fact, it dilates more widely at the times of the menstrual flow." Galen notes (*ibid.* p. 235) that upon the death of the fetus, the os uteri "at once opens up to the extent which is necessary for the foetus to make its exit." He describes the work of the uterus in parturition as follows: "The os opens, whilst the whole fundus approaches as near as possible to the os, expelling the embryo as it does so; and along with the fundus the contiguous parts—which form as it were a girdle round the whole organ—co-operate in the work; they squeeze upon the embryo and propel it bodily outwards."

[2] Literally: the chorion.

3[68]. "A midwife's stool," in order that the laboring woman may be placed in position upon it. In the middle of the stool and in the part where they [3] give support one must have cut out a crescent-shaped cavity of medium size, neither too big so that the woman sinks down to the hips, nor, on the contrary, narrow so that the vagina is compressed. The latter is the more troublesome, for the excessively wide hole can be filled up, if she [4] puts pieces of cloth between. And the entire width of the whole stool must be sufficient to accommodate relatively fleshy women too; and its height medium, for in women of small size a footstool placed beneath makes up the deficiency. Concerning the area below the seat, the sides should be completely closed in with boards, whereas the front and the rear should be open for use in midwifery, as will be related. Concerning the area above, on the sides there should be two parts shaped like the letter Π for the crossbar on which to press the hands in straining. And behind there should be a back, so that both the loins and hips may meet with resistance to any gradual slipping; for if they reclined even with a woman standing behind, by the crooked position they would hinder the movement of the fetus in a straight line.[5] To the lower parts of the stool some people, however, affix a projecting axle which has windlasses on each side and a knob, so that in extractions of the fetus [6] they may place nooses or ropes circularly round the arms or other parts of the fetus, attach the ends to the knob and effect the extraction

[3] I.e. the midwives.

[4] I.e. the midwife whose property the chair was and who brought it along to the house where the delivery took place; cf. Diepgen, p. 179.

[5] It was, apparently, believed desirable that the pelvic region remain in a vertical position to allow the fetus to descend vertically. A solid back would more efficiently oppose any deviation brought about by the tendency of the parturient to slip than would the mere support by an attendant.

[6] I.e. extraction by hooks of a fetus that cannot be delivered alive. On this procedure cf. book IV, ch. III.

<by> rotation—not knowing the general rule that extraction of the fetus in difficult labor must take place with the woman lying down.[7] The stool then must be such as we have said, or it must be a chair, cut out in front or also in back.[8] . . .

And "two beds"[9]: one made up softly for rest after delivery and the other hard for lying down during delivery, lest on a worn-out bed[10] <the loins give way with the sagging of the bed> . . . <and one must make the woman lie down> on her back, the feet drawn together, the thighs separated, while something is placed under the hips, so that the vagina inclines downwards.

III. <*What Must One Do in Delivery?*>

4[69]. . . . and one must first soothe the pains by touching with warm hands, and afterwards drench pieces of cloth with warm, sweet olive oil and put them over the abdomen as well as the labia and keep them saturated with the warm oil for some time, and one must also place bladders filled with warm oil alongside. When the orifice of the uterus opens, the midwife, having first anointed her hands with warm oil, should

[7] Cf. IV, 9.

[8] A sentence has here been omitted which is so corrupt that no attempt at translating it has been made.

[9] Cf. above, p. 70.

[10] Further details about the beds and the discussion of "the proper room" are lost in the Greek original. But the main points seem indicated by Caelius Aurelianus (*Gynaecia*, p. 34, 869 ff.). "The bed should also be low, so that the midwife when sitting can restrain the parturient. Also it should be solidly located, lest it shake when the fetus is drawn down. And the place in which delivery takes place and where the women rest after delivery should be of medium size. Indeed a small room makes people suffocate and a big one is not easily found warm. Besides, the air should be of moderate temperature; for cold air by its contrast has a somewhat astringent action; while heat greatly diminishes the strength of the parturient."

insert the forefinger of the left hand, the nail of which has been cut short, and first dilate the orifice gently and gradually so that the accessible part of the chorion falls forth, while with the right hand, she should anoint the region with oil—bewaring of such oil as has been used for cooking. And when the accessible part of the chorion attains the size <of an egg> below the orifice of the uterus, if the gravida is weak and toneless one must deliver her lying down since this way is less painful and causes less fear. If, however, she happens to be strong, one must make her get up <and> place her on the so-called midwife's stool . . . one must warm her thoroughly with warm oil and give an instillation of it to prevent easy chilling of the gravida. There should also be laid upon her feet as a covering . . .[11]

5[70a]. There should be three woman helpers, capable of gently allaying the anxiety of the gravida even if they do not happen to have had experience with birth. Two of them should be at the sides and one behind holding the parturient woman so that she may not sway with <the> pains. But if the midwife's stool is not at hand, the same arrangement can also be made if she sits on a woman's lap. However, the woman must be robust, that she may bear the weight of the woman sitting

[11] From a comparison with Muscio I, 64, it would seem as if a lengthy passage were missing in which Soranus opposed the woman's walking about, washing, and partaking of food as recommended by the older physicians. Galen (*On the Natural Faculties* III, 3; p. 235 f.) gives the following account: "The midwife, however, does not make the parturient woman get up at once and sit down on the . . . chair, but she begins by palpating the os as it gradually dilates, and the first thing she says is that it has dilated 'enough to admit the little finger,' then that 'it is bigger now,' and as we make enquiries from time to time, she answers that the size of the dilatation is increasing. And when it is sufficient to allow of the transit of the foetus, she then makes the patient get up from her bed and sit on the chair, and bids her make every effort to expel the child." This account makes it clear that the attending physician relied on the midwife to make the manual examination.

upon her and be able to hold her firmly during the pangs of labor. Moreover the midwife, after having covered herself properly with an apron above and below, should sit down opposite and below the laboring woman; for the extraction of the fetus must take place from a higher towards a lower plane. But to make her kneel, as some have deemed good, renders it both difficult to work and undignified; and the same is true of having her stand, as Heron required, in a pit so that her hands might not work from above, for this is not only awkward but also impossible in second-floor rooms. Therefore, the midwife, with legs parted and bending the left one forward a little to make it easy to work with the left hand, should sit down and, as has been said, in front of the laboring woman. For the lower sides of the stool, as we advised,[12] should be blocked in, while the rear is occupied by the assistant for necessary service; for by placing a pledget underneath she must restrain the anus of the gravida because of the prolapses and ruptures which occur in straining. Furthermore it is proper that the face of the gravida should be visible to the midwife who shall allay her anxiety, assuring her that there is nothing to fear and that delivery will be easy.

6[70b]. Next, one must advise her to drive her breath into the flanks without screaming, rather with groaning and detention of the breath. For some inexperienced women, keeping the breath in the upper parts and not driving it downwards have brought about a tumor of the bronchus.[13] Whence, for the unhindered passage of the breath, it is necessary to loosen their girdles as well as to free the chest of any binder,

[12] Cf. above, p. 71.

[13] The Greek term is "bronchokēlē" which is defined by the Pseudo-Galenic "Medical Definitions" (ed. Kühn, vol. 19, p. 443) as: "Bronchokēlē is a tumor around the throat, different in its constitution from that in the scrotum." It is, therefore, possible that Soranus thought of goiter.

though not on account of the vulgar conception [14] according to which womenfolk are unwilling to suffer any fetter and thus <also> loosen the hair; it is rather for the above-mentioned reason [15] that even loosening the hair possibly effects good tonus of the head. Thus one must advise the women to compress their breath and not to give in to the pains, but to strain themselves most when they are present.

The midwife should beware of fixing her gaze steadfastly on the genitals of the laboring woman, lest being ashamed, her body become contracted. And with a circular movement of her finger the midwife should dilate the orifice of the uterus <and> the labia [16] . . .

. . . and her [17] orifice rises straight up, but sometimes it

[14] Viz., that any constriction impedes labor.

[15] I.e. free passage of the breath.

[16] Here a lacuna of 30⅕ lines follows, where the subsequent passage from Caelius Aurelianus and Muscio (Caelius Aurelianus, *Gynaecia,* p. 35, 903 ff.) found its place: "If the bag (i.e. the chorion) is not ruptured at all, it should be opened with an ointment and if it has opened spontaneously [the ointment should be used] to widen the opening. At the same time the midwife should take care in case the orifice is open, lest the fetus fall down suddenly and be broken by the impact and lest the distention cause the navel cord to be ruptured, when the flow of blood will endanger the patient. When the bag is sufficiently open, the head of the fetus is driven out next; for thus it is carried when nature fulfills her duty properly. And the birth is even more favorable when [the fetus] descends with its face turned downwards. Then one need assist the uterine orifice only with slight stretching, so that the head may come out more easily; in addition, one should take care that it be not pressed and thereby receive serious damage.

But when the head has issued, the orifice of the uterus should also be distended lest it close by natural necessity and choke the infant. For it constantly varies between these movements so that it now opens, now contracts. When the shoulders have also been born, the infant should be drawn out by the hands of the midwife. And it should not be moved in a straight line, but should rather be inclined somewhat sideways and should be moved by a gentle pull from both sides."

[17] This may refer to any feminine Greek noun, possibly to "uterus," in which case the meaning would be: "and the orifice of the uterus."

points downwards. Now she [18] must insert the fingers gently at the time of dilatation and pull the fetus forward, giving way when the uterus draws itself together, but pulling lightly when it dilates. For to do this at the time of contraction produces inflammation, or hemorrhage of the uterus, or drags it downwards. And the servants standing at the sides should softly press the mass down towards the lower parts with their hands. Finally the midwife herself should receive the infant, having first covered her hands with pieces of cloth or, as those in Egypt do, with scraps of thin papyrus, so that it may neither slip off nor be squeezed, but rest softly. Now if the secundines are extruded at the same time, one should proceed further; if, however, the afterbirth [19] remains behind, the laboring woman should lie down and one ought to put the newborn . . .[20]

. . . . .

[XXII]. ⟨*On Retained Secundines.*⟩ (See p. 196.)

IV [XXIII]. ⟨*What Is the Care of the Woman after Labor?*⟩

. . . . .

[18] This probably refers to the midwife.

[19] Literally: *chorion.*

[20] Here Caelius Aurelianus (*Gynaecia,* p. 36, 925 ff.) seems to continue: ". . . close to her so that it neither stretch the umbilical cord nor cause the danger of rupture. If, however, the mother is sitting, the infant must be put upon a pillow. And the woman must be ordered to expel the secundines by straining while the midwife has her left hand inserted into the uterus before the latter closes and hinders their ejection. Then the parts [i.e. of the secundines] must be grasped at their roots and gently pulled, even if they have receded to the fundus of the uterus and are held there. They should be pulled forth gently in one and the other direction rather than in a straight line, lest the uterus be pulled forth together with them." See also below, book IV, 16.

v[xxv]. *On the Intumescence of the Breasts.*

7[76]. A discussion of the proposed subject also falls under Care of the Woman after Labor. For with the influx of the milk, the breasts swell greatly and at first become heavy; this is called *chondrōsis* (lumpiness); later on they also hurt and become tense and inflamed, and such a state is called *spargēsis* (intumescence). Consequently, one must carry out treatment as against inflammation, and in the beginning one must use mildly contracting things (such as a soft sea sponge moistened in diluted vinegar, with a close-fitting bandage, or tender dates triturated with bread and diluted vinegar); but if one wishes to dry up the milk, one must also use alum, or fleawort and coriander, or purslane. If, however, swelling has set in with tension or clotting, the breasts should be poulticed with relaxing poultices (e.g. bread well softened by a mixture of water and olive oil or hydromel; or linseed and wheat or fenugreek with hydromel). If, however, the breasts cannot stand the weight one should first apply fomentations and press them[21] down while soaking them with sweet warm olive oil; the fomenting should be done with sea sponges squeezed in warm water or in a decoction of fenugreek or mallow or linseed.[22] ⟨But⟩ if suppuration has set in one must empty the fluid as we have shown in the books on "Surgery." And when the inflammation is past its height, one must apply wax salve only.

[21] I.e. the breasts.

[22] The text of this whole sentence is very doubtful and the meaning not quite clear. Caelius Aurelianus (*Gynaecia,* p. 39, 993 ff.) reads: "At si forte mamme pondus ferre non poterint, adhibenda fomenta ex oleo dulci calido prostrata molli limpida lana. tunc etiam spongiis aqua calida expressis partes vaporande, vel decoctione fenugreci, radicum malve, lini seminis aut hibisci."

8[77]. If, however, the mother is not going to nurse the newborn herself, one must also mix a certain amount of properly ground pyrite, then apply the breast binder which is gradually tightened; for when the vessels collapse the influx is hindered, and thus the milk runs dry; if it does not, one must be more liberal in the application of heat and close-fitting bandages. One should not, however, allow the breasts to be sucked at the first discomfort, as if sucking, due to the secretion of the <milk>, relieves the tension; for quite on the contrary, more milk streams into the parts in proportion to the sensation [23] of being sucked, and the nipples are irritated in proportion to their being bruised. One must also beware of fomenting with brine, with a mixture of vinegar and brine, and with sea water, for the inflammation is aggravated by their pungency. Some women, however, anoint the breasts with cyperus together with wine and saffron, some with henna oil and triturated pumice stone, some with cummin together with water or oil, <or> with moist alum together with vinegar and rose oil to the consistency of honey. Other women poultice with cummin together with raisins from which the stones have been removed, or with sesame together with honey; others with green tribulus boiled in vinegar, or with ivy or dried figs or bran boiled in the same manner; and when clotting has set in,[24] with celery or peppermint or cabbage together with bread. But of these things one must reject the pungent ones entirely, and of the others one should adopt the mildly astringent ones in the beginning and the gently relaxing ones in the subsequent period. Such, then, is the treatment of the

[23] Sensation probably connotes not only the actual feeling on the part of the woman but also the stimulus for the increase in the supply of milk.
[24] Cf. above, p. 77.

woman in childbed; how to care for the newborn has to be taken up next.

ON THE CARE OF THE NEWBORN.

9[78]. The subject of rearing children is broad and manifold. For it comprises the consideration as to: which of the offspring is worth rearing, how one should sever the navel cord and swaddle and cleanse the infant which is to be reared, in what manner one should bathe it, how one should bed it and what kind of a nurse one should select, and which milk is best and what one should do if it gives out, and when and how one should wean the newborn; teething, and the mishaps which at times befall them. But lest the matter become difficult to treat, we shall present the whole in the form of short single summaries.

VI[XXVI]. *How to Recognize the Newborn That Is Worth Rearing.*

10[79]. Now the midwife, having received the newborn, should first put it upon the earth,[25] having examined beforehand whether the infant is male or female, and should make an announcement by signs as is the custom of women. She

[25] The putting of the newborn upon the ground (actually earth?) corresponded to a custom prevalent in Rome and among the Teutonic peoples. The German term *Hebamme* (midwife) is said to be derived from the midwife's duty of picking up the infant from the ground and handing it over to the father. Cf. *Encyclopaedia of Religion and Ethics,* ed. James Hastings, vol. II, New York, Scribner's, 1910, pp. 649 and 662.

should also consider whether it is worth rearing or not. And the infant which is suited by nature for rearing will be distinguished by the fact that its mother has spent the period of pregnancy in good health, for conditions which require medical care, especially those of the body, also harm the fetus and enfeeble the foundations of its life. Second, by the fact that it has been born at the due time, best at the end of nine months, and if it so happens, later; but also after only seven months. Furthermore by the fact that when put on the earth it immediately cries with proper vigor; for one that lives for some length of time without crying, or cries but weakly, is suspected of behaving so on account of some unfavorable condition. Also by the fact that it is perfect in all its parts, members and senses; that its ducts, namely of the ears, nose, pharynx, urethra, anus are free from obstruction; that the natural functions of every <member> are neither sluggish nor weak; that the joints bend and stretch; that it has due size and shape and is properly sensitive in every respect. This we may recognize from pressing the fingers against the surface of the body, for it is natural to suffer pain from everything that pricks or squeezes. And by conditions contrary to those mentioned, the infant not worth rearing is recognized.

vii[xxvii]. *How to Sever the Navel Cord.*

11[80]. When the newborn has rested a little after the shaking caused by the birth, one should lift it up and perform the omphalotomy. One must cut off the navel cord at a distance of four fingerbreadths from the abdomen, by means of something sharp-edged, that no bruising may arise. And of all material, iron cuts best; but the majority of the women practising midwifery approve of the section by means of glass, a reed, a potsherd, or the thin crust of bread; or by forcefully squeezing it apart with a cord, since during the earliest period, cutting with iron is deemed of ill omen. This is absolutely ridiculous, <for> crying itself is of ill omen, and yet it is with this that the child begins its life. And lest a sympathetic affection and irritation arise, when this part of the body [26] is sawn through or crushed on all sides, it is better to be less superstitious and rather cut the navel cord [27] with a knife. Then one must squeeze out what is contained in it, which is nothing but coagulated blood, and must next ligate the cut end tightly, e.g. with a twisted piece of wool or with a thread of the warp or a strand of wool or something similar; for a linen cord cuts into the soft body and causes pain which is hard to bear. To ligate the part, as we have indicated, is necessary, however, lest danger of hemorrhage arise, since the vessels here served to convey the blood and pneuma from the gravida to the body of the infant. For this reason, after the section some have cauterized the navel cord [27] by means of a heated pipe or broad part of the knife. We refuse to do this, for cauterized parts undergo great pain and vehement inflammation. If, however, the afterbirth [28] has not been removed, one must ligate the cord [29] in two places and then cut between, so that by the one ligature we may prevent hemorrhage of the newborn and by the other, hemorrhage of the mother, for the afterbirth [30] is still attached to her.

[26] The navel cord is obviously considered a part of the infant's body.

[27] Literally: *omphalos*.

[28] Literally: *chorion*.

[29] Literally: *ourachos*. It seems that in this section Soranus uses the terms navel (*omphalos*) and urachus interchangeably for the umbilical cord.

[30] See note 28.

VIII[XXVIII]. ⟨*How to Cleanse.*⟩

12[81]. After omphalotomy, the majority of the barbarians, as the Germans and Scythians, and even some of the Hellenes, put the newborn into cold water in order to make it firm [31] and to let die, as not worth rearing, one that cannot bear the chilling but becomes livid or convulsed. And others wash it with wine mixed with brine, others with pure wine, others with the urine of an innocent child, while others sprinkle it with fine myrtle or with oak gall. We, however, reject all of these. For cold, on account of its strong and sudden condensing action the like of which the child has not experienced, harms all; and though the harm resulting from the cold escapes notice in those more resistant it is, on the other hand, demonstrated by those susceptible to disease when they are seized by convulsions and apoplexies. Certainly, the fact that the child did not withstand the injury does not prove that it was impossible for it to live if unharmed; more resistant children will also thrive better if not harmed in any way. And if there is any need of cooling, the cooling effect of the air will be sufficient, on account of which the newborn immediately cries since it is affected by the unaccustomed cold, having just come forth from the warm and enfolding uterus. The wine, on the other hand, because of its effluvia, overpowers and causes stupor not only ⟨in⟩ children who are so tender but also in those already full-grown; and the urine

[31] Aristotle, "Politica" VII, 17; 1336a 12–18: "To accustom children to the cold from their earliest years is also an excellent practice, which greatly conduces to health, and hardens them for military service. Hence many barbarians have a custom of plunging their children at birth into a cold stream; others, like the Celts, clothe them in a light wrapper only" (Aristotle, *Oxford transl.*).

likewise, because it is ill-smelling. And myrtle and oak gall, although astringent, do not cleanse; yet there is need of things which both cleanse and have an astringent action, that the natural crust of sticky blood on the body be removed, and at the same time the surface be hardened and rendered immune against the development of rashes.

13[82]. Therefore the following method of sprinkling with salt might be acceptable. Taking fine and powdery salt, or natron or aphronitre, one must besprinkle the newborn, watching out for the eyes and the mouth; for if it enters these parts it produces ulceration and severe inflammation or suffocation. Nor should one besprinkle with much salt, for by too great pungency the physique, which is still tender and very weak, is corroded; nor with little, since the surface is not rendered sufficiently firm. But the newborn being delicate, it may be necessary to beat up the salt with honey or with olive oil <or> with the juice of barley or fenugreek or mallow. After having cleansed the body, one must bathe it with lukewarm water and wash away all the covering emulsion.[32] Then one must do the same a second time: besprinkle with salt, but wash off with much warmer water. And with the fingers one must squeeze out the thick mucus which lies in the nose, and clear the mouth as well as the auditory canals, and one must also treat the eyes by an injection of olive oil; for it is good thus to wash off the thickest moisture in them; if this is not done, in most cases the nurslings become dim-sighted. With the little finger whose nail has first been cut short one must for the unhindered passing of the excrements dilate the anus and divide the thin and membranous

[32] The Greek word indicates a soapy emulsion; it is probably the product of the cleansing substance and the *vernix caseosa,* the unctuous substance covering the infant.

body which often is grown round it. Forthwith, what is usually called meconium is excreted. And to the umbilicus one must apply a little piece of lint soaked in oil, or a piece of wool, but must reject cummin since it is pungent. Now of the navel cord [33] left behind, some have attached the ligated part to the thigh; but it is better to bend it double, wrap around a lock of wool and place it gently in the middle of the umbilicus; for if in addition it is pressed down by the weight, this part will soon be moulded into a better-shaped cavity.

IX[XXIX]. ⟨*How to Swaddle.*⟩

14[83]. After the sprinkling with salt and the ablution, one must swaddle the newborn. Now Antigenes, adopting the swaddling which is called Thessalian, throws a mattress filled with hay or chaff into a hollowed oblong log, he then spreads out a piece of cloth and lays the newborn upon it covered as far as the loins with rags and bandages; then, in addition he ties it fast with swaddling bands which are passed through notches, which the log must have at its sides. But this method of bandaging is hard to endure and cruel. Rather one must mould every part according to its natural shape, ⟨and⟩ if something has been twisted during the time of delivery, one must correct it and bring it into its natural shape; if, however, some part has been squeezed and has become swollen, one must anoint it with white lead triturated with water, or with litharge. The midwife should put the newborn down gently on her lap which has been covered entirely with wool or with a piece of cloth so that the infant may not cool down when laid bare while every part is swaddled. Then she must

[33] Literally: *omphalos.*

take soft woolen bandages which are clean and not too worn out, some of them three fingers in breadth, others four fingers. "Woolen," because of the smoothness of the material and because linen ones shrink from the sweat; "soft," so as not to cause bruises when covering the body which is still delicate; "clean," so that they may be light and not heavy, nor of evil smell, nor irritate the surface by containing natron; and "not too worn out": for whereas new ones are heavy, worn out ones are too cold, and sometimes rough as well and very easily torn. They must have neither hems nor selvages, otherwise they cut or compress unevenly: some parts more, others less. They must be of medium breadth, for the narrow ones cut, while the broad ones do not compress, but wrinkle; and "three as well as four fingers" wide in order that the former may fit the limbs, the latter the thorax.

15[84]. The midwife then should take the end of the bandage, put it over its hand and, winding it round, carry it over the extended fingers; then over the middle of the hand, the forearm and the upper arm, slightly compressing the parts at the wrist but keeping the rest up to the armpit loose. Having also swaddled the other arm in the same manner, she should then wrap one of the broader bandages circularly around the thorax, exerting an even pressure when swaddling males, but in females binding the parts at the breasts more tightly, yet keeping the region of the loins loose, for in women this form is more becoming. After this one must swaddle each leg separately, for to join them naked and bind them up together is apt to produce ulceration; for the juxtaposition of bodies which are as yet soft makes them quickly burn with inflammation. The midwife must wind the bandage to the very tips of the toes, keep the region of the thighs and the calves loose, but tighten the parts at the knees and their hollows as well as the instep and the ankles, so that the ends of the feet be broadened but their middle be contracted. Afterwards she should lay the arms along the sides and the feet one against the other, and with a broad bandage she should wrap up the whole infant circularly from the thorax to the feet; since if the hands are put inside the wrapping, they become accustomed to extension. For the confinement of the joints for any length of time is apt to thicken the sinews [34] (so as even to bring about ankylosis) ; however, by wrapping up the little hands just at first, they are prevented from becoming twisted by inordinate movements. Also, putting the fingers to the eyes, often causes impaired vision. Now between the ankles, the knees, and the elbows too, a piece of wool should be inserted so that the prominences may not be ulcerated by the relatively forcible pressure and juxtaposition of the parts. The little head should be covered by bandaging it circularly with a soft clean cloth or piece of wool.

It is also possible first to put a long broad cloth or piece of wool beneath the back; then after the swaddling mentioned before (omitting the one external bandage which all parts have in common) one must first fold the underlying cloth or piece of wool over the upper parts below the neck, then over the whole child except the head; afterwards one must wrap the whole newborn around with a broader bandage about five fingers in breadth, covering the head, however, as we have shown.

Another possibility is to put two pieces of cloth underneath, so that one is of good size and capable of embracing the whole body, the other one large enough for the reception of the faeces, to go around the loins only. For, as we have said before, one should not, because it is too burdensome, cover

[34] Literally: "nerves" (*neura*).

the thorax together with the abdomen with clean wool yet leave the other parts <un>covered.

x[xxx]. *On Laying the Newborn Down.*

16[85]. Then one must lay the newborn down, but not on something hard and resistant as do the Thracians and Macedonians who tie down the newborn on a level board, so that the part around the neck and the back of the head may be flattened (for thus it happens that the bodies are ulcerated and bruised because of the roughness beneath, and the head made ugly; besides, even if this form were becoming, it could be accomplished without danger or sympathetic involvement by shaping during the bath). <Nor> must one lay it down upon anything too soft lest this be very yielding and thus, again, the backbone or the neck be distorted. In fact, the newborn should be bedded avoiding either extreme, for instance upon a pillow filled with flock or, otherwise, with soft hay; and the mattress should be hollowed out like a channel, so that the newborn when put down should <not> roll about. And the little head should be placed in a somewhat raised position, on which account some people, not unreasonably, permit bedding in troughs which have been made up as beds. The coverlets should be warmer or thinner according to the season, and what lies underneath should be aired and changed piece by piece, so as not to chill the newborn nor to make it full of evil smell. This is why some people have also strewn sweet bay or myrtle leaves underneath to give a sweet smell; others, however, avoiding the sweet smell itself as overpowering have rejected them. The room must be clean and moderately warm and must have neither too powerful effluvia nor too much light; besides, it is fitting to have plenty of ventilation and to have mosquito nets put up.

XI[XXXI]. ⟨*On Food.*⟩

17[86]. Now after putting the newborn to bed ⟨subsequent to⟩ the swaddling, one must let it rest and, in most cases, abstain from all food up to as long as two days. For it is still violently upset in all parts and its whole body is yet full of maternal food which it ought to digest first, so as at the proper time to take other food readily. That is unless the appetite indicate an earlier time; and in what manner this is to be recognized, we shall show later. After the interval, one must give food to lick: not butter (for being heavy and bad for the stomach it does harm), nor southernwood with butter (for this, too, is too pungent and upsetting) nor nosesmart or kneaded barley meal (for the nosesmart is pungent, and the barley, which roughens, produces inflammation and in any case scratches the gullet). Instead, one ought to give honey moderately boiled (for raw it causes flatulence and is pungent, and overboiled it is more astringent, whereas boiled down correctly it mildly purges the stomach and the bowel). One must gently anoint the mouth of the newborn with the finger, and must then drop lukewarm hydromel into it; for in this way what is raw and thick in substance is made fine, the appetite becomes related to its memory, the gullet is opened, by permeation and purgation of the ducts the way is prepared for the distribution of food ⟨and⟩ the physique is nourished.

18[87]. From the second day on after the treatment, one should feed with milk from somebody well able to serve as a wet nurse, as for twenty days [35] the maternal milk is in most cases unwholesome, being thick, too caseous, and therefore hard to digest, raw, and not prepared to perfection. Furthermore, it is produced by bodies which are in a bad state, agitated and changed to the extent that we see the body altered after delivery when, from having suffered a great discharge of blood, it is dried up, toneless, discolored, and in the majority of cases feverish as well. For all these reasons, it is absurd to prescribe the maternal milk until the body enjoys stable health.

Therefore, one ought to censure Damastes, who orders the mother to give the newborn the breast immediately, contending that it is to this end that nature too has provided for the production of milk beforehand so that the newborn may have food straightway. And one must also blame those who follow his opinion in these things, like Apollonius called Biblas, for by plausible sophistry they attempt to confuse clear evidence. If, however, a woman well able to provide milk is not at hand, during the first three days one must use the honey alone,[36] or mix goats' milk with it. Then one must supply the mother's milk, the first portion having been sucked out beforehand by some stripling (for it is heavy), or squeezed out gently with the hands, since the thick part is hard to suck out and also apt to clog up in newborn children on account of the softness of their gums. But if the circumstances allow a choice of women able to suckle, one

[35] This reading of the ms. which has "twenty days" seems to be correct, although modern editors have changed it to mean "three" days. But "twenty" days is confirmed by Soranus' advice to choose a wet nurse who has had milk for 2 or 3 months (cf. below, p. 94). It is true, he permits maternal milk from the fourth day on, but only if no suitable wet nurse is available. Caelius Aurelianus (or Muscio?) moreover also reads "Maternum enim lac usque ad xx dies est separandum" (*Gynaecia,* p. 44, 1121).

[36] Cf. above, p. 88.

must select the best, and not necessarily the mother, unless she also shows the attributes characteristic of the best nurses. To be sure, other things being equal, it is better to feed the child with maternal milk; for this is more suited to it, and the mothers become more sympathetic towards the offspring, and it is more natural to be fed from the mother after parturition just as before parturition. But if anything prevents it one must choose the best wet nurse, lest the mother grow prematurely old, having spent herself through the daily suckling. For just as <the earth> is exhausted by producing crops after sowing and therefore becomes barren of more, the same happens with the woman who nurses the infant; she either grows prematurely old having fed one child, or the expenditure for the nourishment of the offspring necessarily makes her own body quite emaciated. Consequently, the mother will fare better with a view to her own recovery and to further childbearing, if she is relieved of having her breasts distended too. For as vegetables are sown by gardeners into one soil to sprout and are transplanted into different soil for quick development, lest one soil suffer by both, in the same way the newborn, too, is apt to become more vigorous if borne by one woman but fed by another, in case the mother, by some affliction, is hindered from supplying the food.

XII[XXXII]. *On the Selection of a Wet Nurse.*

19[88]. One should choose a wet nurse not younger than twenty nor older than forty years, who has already given birth twice or thrice, who is healthy, of good habitus, of large frame, and of a good color. Her breasts should be of medium size, lax, soft and unwrinkled, the nipples neither big nor too small and neither too compact nor too porous and discharging milk overabundantly. She should be self-controlled, sympathetic and not ill-tempered, a Greek, and tidy. And for each of these points the reasons are as follows:

She should be in her prime because younger women are ignorant in the rearing of children and their minds are still somewhat careless and childish; while older ones yield a more watery milk because of the atony of the body. In women in their prime, however, every natural function is at its highest. "She should already have given birth twice or thrice," because women with their first child are as yet unpractised in the rearing of children and have breasts whose structure is still infantile, small and too compact; while those who have delivered often have nursed children often and, being wrinkled, produce thin milk which is not at its best. <"Healthy": because healthful> and nourishing <milk> comes from a healthy body, unwholesome and worthless milk from a sickly one; just as water which flows through worthless soil is itself rendered worthless, spoiled by the qualities of its basin. And "she should be of good habitus," that is, fleshy and strong, not only for the same reason, but also lest she easily become too weak for hard work and nightly duties with the result that the milk also deteriorates. "Of large frame": for everything else being equal, milk from large bodies is more nourishing. And "of a good color": for in such women, bigger vessels carry the material up to the breasts so that there is more milk. And "her breasts should be of medium size": for small ones have little milk, whereas excessively large ones have more than is necessary so that if after nursing the surplus is retained it will be drawn out by the newborn when no longer fresh, and in some way already spoiled. If, on the other hand, it is all sucked out by other children or even other animals,[37] <the> wet nurse will be completely exhausted. Besides, the bigger breasts also weigh heavy when they fall upon the nursling; some people even are of the opinion that <such breasts> often have less milk because the food which is brought to them is spent for the increase of their flesh and not for the amount of milk. "Lax and soft and not wrinkled" and having neither a network of visible vessels nor clotted concretions suspended in them. For the breasts which are compact, hard, and have a network of vessels produce little milk; those which are shriveled and wrinkled as in old and thin bodies make it watery, while those which have clotted concretions make it thick and somewhat uneven. "Nipples which are neither big nor small": <for> the big ones bruise the gums and hinder the tongue from co-operation in swallowing, while small ones are difficult to seize and <make> the milk <come out> in small amounts for the sucklings. Therefore, the newborn suffers in suckling and is usually afflicted with so-called *aphthai*.[38] "Neither compact nor too porous and giving forth milk overabundantly": for if they have narrow ducts they do not easily bring forth the milk without being squeezed; consequently in suckling the newborn suffers, since not as much milk is furnished as it is eager to obtain. If, on the other hand, <they> are too porous, they bring on the danger of suffocation, for in suckling the milk is brought to the mouth overabundantly. And the wet nurse should be "self-controlled" so as to abstain from coitus, drinking, lewdness, and any other such pleasure and incontinence. For coitus cools the affection toward <the> nursling by the diversion of sexual pleasure and moreover spoils and dimin-

[37] This seems to suggest that young animals were sometimes employed to empty the breasts.

[38] I.e. thrush; cf. book II, 51.

ishes the milk or suppresses it entirely by stimulating menstrual catharsis through the uterus or by bringing about conception. In regard to drinking, first the wet nurse is harmed in soul as well as in body and for this reason the milk also is spoiled. Secondly, seized by a sleep from which she is hard to awaken, she leaves the newborn untended or even falls down upon it in a dangerous way. Thirdly, too much wine passes its quality to the milk and therefore the nursling becomes sluggish and comatose and sometimes even afflicted with tremor, apoplexy, and convulsions, just as suckling pigs become comatose and stupefied when the sow has eaten dregs. "Sympathetic" and affectionate, that she may fulfill her duties without hesitation and without murmuring. For some wet nurses are so lacking in sympathy towards the nursling that they not only pay no heed when it cries for a long time, but do not even arrange its position when it lies still; rather, they leave it in one position so that often because of the pressure the sinewy parts [39] suffer and consequently become numb and bad. "And not ill-tempered": since by nature the nursling becomes similar to the nurse and accordingly grows sullen if the nurse is ill-tempered, but of mild disposition if she is even-tempered. Besides, angry women are like maniacs and sometimes when the newborn cries from fear and they are unable to restrain it, they let it drop from their hands or overturn it dangerously. For the same reason the wet nurse should not be superstitious and prone to ecstatic states so that she may not expose the infant to danger when led astray by fallacious reasoning, sometimes even trembling like mad. And the wet nurse should be tidy-minded lest the odor of the swaddling clothes cause the

[39] The Greek term *neurōdes* probably here refers to nerves, tendons, and ligaments alike.

child's stomach to become weak and it lie awake on account of itching or suffer some ulceration subsequently. And she should be a Greek so that the infant nursed by her may become accustomed to the best speech.

20[89]. At the most she should have had milk for two or three months. For very early milk, as we have said, is thick of particles and is hard to digest, while late milk is not nutritious, and is thin. But some people say that a woman who is going to feed a male must have given birth to a male, if a female, on the other hand, to a female. One should pay no heed to these people, for they do not consider that mothers of twins, the one being male and the other female, feed both with one and the same milk. And in general, each kind of animal makes use of the same nourishment, male as well as female; and this is ⟨no⟩ reason at all for the male to become more feminine or for the female to become more masculine. One should, on the other hand, provide several wet nurses for children who are to be nursed safely and successfully. For it is precarious for the nursling to become accustomed to one nurse who might become ill or die, and then, because of the change of milk, the child sometimes suffers from the strange milk and is distressed, while sometimes it rejects it altogether and succumbs to hunger.

XIII[XXXIII.] *On Testing the Milk.*

21[90]. One must, however, also examine the milk itself attentively that it may be the best. This is attested first by the fact that the wet nurse is the kind we have described as the best. Secondly, by the fact that the child being nursed by her is in good physical condition. Yet, although it is a sign of suitable milk if the child fed on it is in good physical condition, it does not follow, on the other hand, that an ill-developed child, as one might suppose, is a sign of worthless milk. For it is possible that the milk is suitable but the child is prevented by some disease from being well nourished. For adults too who are sick become ill-nourished though they partake of the best food, the body spoiling what might be nourishing, just as vessels for vinegar spoil the wine that is poured into them, even if it is the best.

22[91]. Thirdly, from the properties of the milk: color, smell, composition, density, the character of its taste and its relative lack of change with time. "Color": if it is a medium white. For livid or greenish milk is spoiled, chalky milk is thick and hard to digest, while red-yellow milk is raw [40] and not brought to perfection and therefore displays a blood-like color. "Smell": ⟨if⟩ it is pleasant. For it ought to have neither an evil, foul, dreg-like, or vinegar-like smell, since all such milk has unhealthy juices. "Composition": ⟨if⟩ it is smooth and even and homogeneous. For if it is stringy and has red or flesh-like streaks, it is raw. "Density" and thickness: if it is moderately dense. For free-running, thin, and watery milk is not nutritious and is apt to disturb the bowels; whereas thick and caseous milk is hard to digest and, similarly to food that has been chewed partially, it blocks up the ducts and, occupying the principal passages, it entails danger to life. Uneven milk, on the other hand, has the injurious effects of both thin and thick milk. ⟨And⟩ moderately thick milk will be recognized by the fact that if a drop is made to fall on the finger nail or a leaf of sweet bay or on something else of similar smoothness, it spreads gently and when rocked

[40] I.e. the body of the wet nurse has not let it undergo the proper physiological "cooking."

it retains, as it were, the same form. <For> milk which runs off immediately is watery, whereas milk that stays together like honey and remains motionless is thick. And the same conclusion is drawn from the fact that the milk on being dropped into twice the amount of water stays the same for a little while and is afterwards dissolved, remaining white to the last. For milk which dissolves immediately is watery, and it is worse if it is reduced into fibrous streaks like water in which meat has been washed, for such milk is also raw. But milk which does not disperse for some length of time and settles, so that when the water is poured off it is found as a caseous substance all around the bottom, is thick and hard to digest. "By the character of its taste": if it is sweet and pleasant to the taste. For milk which is slightly pungent or tastes like vinegar or is bitter or salty or harsh and when dropped into the eyes appears somewhat pungent is bad. "By its relative lack of change with time": the best milk is that which does not turn sour quickly when stored and produces extremely little or no whey, for such milk is nutritious; while milk which easily becomes sour when stored and which produces much whey, is not nutritious. Foamy milk is also bad, for it causes flatulence; and the froth on the surface of the fluid even becomes blown into bubbles when it comes in contact with much air. Sometimes, however, this is a sign of thickness and this will be determined by the fact that the ensuing bubbles last for some time, probably since the air is prevented from evaporating quickly because of the thickness of the milk.

23[92]. But in addition the question is asked, at what time one should test the milk. The majority say: when no error in regimen has been committed by the wet nurse, when her digestion has been good, when she has slept sufficiently, and has eliminated waste material, when her stomach is still empty, and when she has not taken a dose of a drug. For as a result of a faulty regimen, milk which is naturally good seems bad, since it is changed for a while, just as the breath of those suffering from indigestion becomes temporarily but not permanently ill-smelling. On the contrary, however, some people say: after a faulty regimen,[41] since the best milk is that which is not spoiled by anything able to change it for the worse. We, however, examine the milk under both regimens. For the milk which is spoiled by neither regimen is the best; that which does not lose its faults even under a healthy regimen is the worst; while that which changes with the regimen is in between. Therefore <the question arises> as to how to maintain the milk in the best condition.[42]

XIV[XXXIV]. *How to Conduct the Regimen of the Nurse.*

24[93]. No little consideration should be given to the wet nurse so that the newborn may not become ill from spoiled milk nor, owing to the deficiency of milk, the infant pine away and its gullet be harmed by drawing on the nipple for a long time, without, <however,> being able to satisfy its appetite. Consequently, it is proper to avoid idleness and physical inertia (for this makes the milk thick and hard to digest); rather the wet nurse should even take exercise, not of the heavier and athletic type (for this is too hard for women and, since her nutriment is diverted into the good nourishment of her body, the milk decreases steadily) but of

[41] I.e. the milk should be tested after the wet nurse has committed a dietary mistake.

[42] This is the subject of the following section.

a moderate and light sort. Therefore, when she first wakes up from her sleep, she should not rise from the bed immediately, not before she has felt that the food is being digested, that the hypochondriac region is light, the abdomen soft, her eructations empty and neither smoky nor acid. Then having occupied herself with the elimination [43] of waste material, she should go out for a walk, and following this she should also take exercise in a carriage drawn by animals. She should also work her body hard at such exercises as are apt to shake all parts, but particularly those of the hands and shoulders, so that the nourishment may be carried more to these parts. Such exercises are: playing with a ball, especially a hollow one, and throwing light weights; for those who are too poor, however, rowing or drawing up water in a vessel, winnowing and grinding grain, preparing bread, making beds and whatever is done with a certain bending of the body. For the upper parts of the body are exercised more, and the breasts hanging down for some time do not remain idle either and produce more nutritious and more plentiful milk when the nutriment is brought to them abundantly. Therefore it is advantageous always to have them unbound, lest by binding the milk be checked; and especially at the time of the exercise that they may move together with the whole body. After the exercises, on most days she should content herself with anointing alone (for baths make the milk watery). At intervals, however, she should in addition take baths, not in warm water only, but also in cold water together with the warm.

25[94]. As to food, she should forego food that has bad juices, that which is not nourishing and which is hard to digest; while she ought to take food which has good juices,

[43] Literally: "grinding up." The whole elaborate expression may simply mean the emptying of bladder and bowels.

which is nourishing and is easily digestible. In particular, she ought to forego leek and onions, garlic, preserved meat or fish, radish, pulse, and all preserved food (for they make the milk pungent) and most vegetables (for they are watery and not nourishing); and meat of sheep and oxen, and this especially if roasted, for it is bad for the stomach, hard to digest, and makes poor material for the yielding of abundant milk. Rather, she should partake of pure bread, carefully prepared and leavened and made from spring wheat, the yolks of eggs, brain, thrushes, the young of pigeons and domestic birds, fishes living among rocks, bass, red mullet and generally those which are palatable, good for the stomach and of wholesome juices, and the meat of suckling pigs. But she must avoid everything highly spiced and dressed with rich sauce, for, greatly flattering the taste, it produces indigestion by which the milk is poisoned along with the other things in the body. Therefore she must also aim at moderate consumption, so that indigestion does not arise from excessive quantity, and as much is taken as will easily be digested; this especially if sleeplessness occurs on account of her care of the newborn.

26[95]. Furthermore, the wet nurse must partake of the said food according to a definite scheme. For the first seven days, and at most ten, she should take simple and easily digested food like a soup, a porridge which is ⟨not⟩ too fat, eggs, bread, and water as a drink. If possible one should give this even before the first day, since it makes the milk thinner and more digestible. For the newborn needs such milk because, being as yet very tender and having narrow ducts, it offers a difficult passage for milk which is still too thick. But after the first week, till the end of the second or third week, one should also give a little tender fish together with the above food, or the meat of suckling pigs, or brains, so that the milk may become more nourishing. But after the second or third week, that is, when the infant has become firm of body and able to receive more nourishing substances, the wet nurse should also take some medium-sized fowl, later bigger fowl as well, doing so in proportion to the newborn's strength and growth; then she should add the meat of hares or antelopes or kids, and later pork besides; for milk from more nourishing substances is more nourishing. Subsequently, she should partake of various foods, so that the newborn too may be accustomed to their various properties. For the qualities of the food partaken are conveyed also to the milk, and therefore the milk of goats is of unpleasant taste and a little astringent because goats delight in feeding on grass of this character; whereas the milk of sheep is of pleasant taste and sweet because the food of sheep is of the same sort. And she should take water as a drink for at least forty days, and from then on a certain amount of honey wine every second or third day. But when the newborn has become strong and firm of body and has a good color together with a good state of nourishment, she should drink a little wine which is white, clear, not mixed with sea water, moderately tart, and of medium age. At first, however, she should have a drink once every few days, then every third, then every second day; after this daily and not only once, but even twice, later as much as is necessary to quench her thirst. For thus the newborn will be fed without harm by milk affected by wine, whereas in an earlier period it is not adapted by nature to endure such potency without harm.

27[96]. Let no one be at a loss how the child while ⟨within⟩ the uterus before parturition could have endured all the qualities mentioned when its mother partook of wine and various foods. In answer one should say: being controlled at that time by the faculties of the mother, as if it were part of her, it did not fall ill, whereas after parturition, subsisting on its own and having as yet weak functions, it is easily affected by qualities too potent; in the same way slips when still attached to big trees also share the advantage of their rigidity, bear fruit and withstand the onrush of winds, but when separated and planted to subsist on their own are easily harmed by a light breeze. That the wet nurse is not injured by wine now is, therefore, no reason to believe that the infant will not be badly affected either. Rather, one should argue that the wine is stronger than the physique of the newborn and so the majority of those who are fed carelessly are seized by epileptic convulsions.

xv[xxxv]. *What One Should Do if the Milk Stops, or Becomes Spoiled or Thick or Thin.*

28[97]. It the milk decreases and stops, or becomes spoiled or thin or thick, it is good to give the milk of another wet nurse; but if the circumstances do not permit this, one must prescribe a regimen for the present one, lest the newborn fall ill. When, therefore, the milk ceases, one must consider whether this happens because of some local disease of the uterus or of some other organ, or <because> of general atrophy of the whole body, or whether the milk decreases naturally, nature no longer being able to produce as much as is necessary for the suckling. And if some diseased condition can be recognized, one must remove it accordingly, for when the disease is removed the obstacle to the function is removed also. If, however, disease is not the cause, she [44] must take relaxing exercises, walks, and must rub herself and be rubbed by others, at the same time holding her breath; and finally her breasts should also be massaged gently. She should also take vocal exercise, baths, food which has wholesome juices, her mind should be diverted and she should do things that above all are apt to exercise the upper parts. For if thereby the whole body is made to thrive, the parts in the region of the breasts thrive too. Suckling should also be more frequent, for in response to this sensation, more nutriment is provided.

Mnesitheus, however, advises vomiting twice daily, paying no heed to the fact that vomiting results rather in destruction except when one wishes to set a chronic disease aright.[45] And some people have used aromatic potions and little pills, ⟨the⟩ so-called milk pills.[46] They have also given the breasts of those animals to eat, which by nature have much milk. Others have burned owls and bats [47] and have sprinkled their ashes into drinks or smeared them together with some liquid on the breasts. But one must reject each of these things, for they upset the stomach, effect corruption, and will thus double the atrophy.

29[98]. If there is too much milk, the wet nurse should

[44] I.e. the wet nurse.

[45] Soranus here refers to the "cyclic treatment" of chronic diseases as practised by the methodists (cf. Introduction, p. xxxv) which included drastic procedures such as the use of strong emetics. For examples cf. below, p. 159 f.

[46] The composition of these "milk pills" is unknown.

[47] The owl here mentioned is the "little owl" (*Athene noctua*), sacred to Athena. The bird was surrounded by much superstition. Zopyrus, a physician of the first century B.C., among other things recommended owl's brain and the owl itself as ingredients for galactogenous potions (cf. Oribasius, *Collect. med.* XIV, 64; vol. 2, p. 596). Galen (ed. Kühn, vol. 12, p. 258) on the other hand, relates the belief that bat's blood smeared upon girls' breasts keeps them firm.

solidify her body by more vigorous exercises; and if the milk is too thick, she should take baths, eat foods with the consistency of gruel, partake of those things which are not very nourishing, and she should drink water. Some people, however, amongst whom are the followers of Moschion, have given capers, radishes, and preserved meat or fish. One should not agree with them, for even if the thickness of the milk were diluted by the pungent diet, its quality would be spoiled and would become irritating and <do> more <harm>. If, however, the milk has become too thin, one should omit the baths, which have a natural liquefying tendency; but should use for food porridge prepared from far [48] or spelt, eggs that can be sipped, pine cones, pigs' feet, snouts, and ears (for there is something viscous and glutinous in them), the meat of kids, sometimes roasted, sometimes boiled, and a little wine granted that the newborn is far enough developed. But if the milk is spoiled, which in most cases occurs from indigestion, sexual intercourse, and foods with bad juices—one must put an end to each of these and must return to a wholesome and healthy regimen. So much for wet nurses; and now it is necessary to come back to the other things <which> form part of the care of the newborn.

XVI[XXXVI]. *On the Bath and Massage of the Newborn.*

30[99]. One must, indeed, pay rather strict attention to the bath so that the newborn be neither bathed continually nor be much softened by dousing. This is what most women do. For they give it three baths day and night and pour water over it to the point of exhaustion, delighting in the fact that

[48] Probably some kind of spelt.

when it has grown weary after the bath it keeps quiet and falls asleep. But this is harmful, for the body becomes weak, susceptible to disease, easily cooled and easily affected by any harm, and above all, the head is wont to be injured, the senses too. Therefore, one should give it its bath during the daytime, never by night, and not two or three times, except when there is need, when it soils itself very much or is roughened by a rash.

31[100]. The method of bathing and massage is as follows: One must first select a small room which is moderately warm, and must exclude bright light. After the midwife has sat down and spread a linen towel <or> a piece of cloth over her lap and knees, she should then lay the newborn down and, having taken off the swaddling clothes, anoint it with lukewarm olive oil. Next, with her left hand she should hold its right arm under the armpit, so that its breast rest upon her forearm while it is a little inclined toward the right side; and with her right hand she should pour warm water, well-tempered to the pleasure of the newborn. For water that is well-tempered for us is yet too hot for the child because of the extraordinary delicacy of its body. And it will be proper in proportion to add some warm water when the first becomes cool and to pour water over the body till it becomes flushed and evenly warm. Then she must turn the newborn and while it is on its back she should furthermore wash and cleanse its thighs, buttocks, the parts around the neck and armpits (for the dirt clings to them). Then, finally, with her forefinger dipped into pure water or olive oil, she should remove the saliva which is in the mouth, should handle gently the tongue, the gums, and the corners of the mouth and should press lightly the lower abdomen to provoke urination. But after some days the newborn should become accustomed to being washed with tepid water after the warm water, with a view to the practice of cold bathing, which will keep it from becoming easily chilled.

32[101]. After the bath one must grasp the newborn by the ankles and let it hang with the head downwards,[49] in order that the vertebrae may be separated, the spine given the right curves, and the sinews [50] be untangled, so to speak. Then one must gently arrange it upon the lap of the woman who has given the bath and, covering it with the piece of cloth or linen towel which had previously been put under it, wipe it dry. Next, one must anoint freely and at once massage and model every part so that imperceptibly that which is as yet not fully formed is shaped into its natural characteristics. Thus, holding the wrist of the right hand [51] and stretching it out, the wet nurse should now rub in an oblique direction from the left buttock over the spine, then again she should hold the right ankle and rub from the left shoulder blade towards the right leg. Furthermore, she should bend back the limbs towards the spine, moving the tip of the right foot towards the tip of the left hand and the left towards the right. For thus the sinews [52] of the joints are made supple, each ⟨of which⟩ becomes more mobile by the various rotations, and if something viscous has penetrated into the joints while the organism was formed, it is squeezed out. And after making the legs supple, singly, she should bring both legs together, and with one hand she should keep them together and stretch them, while with the other she should rub the whole length.

33[102]. And as to particulars: she should flatten out

[49] This is still being done to remove mucus.

[50] Literally: "nerves" (*neura*).

[51] "Arm" would give a better meaning. For the meaning of *cheir* as "arm" cf. e.g. Galen, *De usu partium* II, 2 (ed. Helmreich, vol. 1, p. 67, 1).

[52] See above, note 50.

the hollows of the knees by applying the ball of the thumb;[53] after the ankles have been brought near to each other she should join and shape them. Massaging from the heels, she should correct the protruding parts higher up by bringing into line what diverges. Then she should bend the legs back, bringing the heels to the buttocks. Furthermore, with the flat of the hand she should smooth out the spine by both straight and circular movements. Then she should make it hollow by pressing upwards along its length with the thumb, from the part between the buttocks to the back of the head, <and again> in a straight line from the neck to the os sacrum, so that the arrangement of the vertebrae may be perfected, and with it comeliness and ease of movement. Afterwards, for the sake of comeliness, she should hollow out the region around the buttocks by pressing with the thumb and forefinger. Furthermore, by applying her clenched fist, she should gently push away the parts overlying the highest vertebra of the spine lest a lordosis[54] arise; and in the same manner down the back and between the shoulders so that these parts may not easily be distorted nor become deformed. Afterwards, she should first, by rotatory movements with each hand, massage the little head round and round. Secondly, with her hands facing each other she should somehow mould it, now with one hand placed against the back of the head and the other against the forehead, now with one against the top of the head and the other under the chin. And she should dexterously bring the skull into good proportions, so that it may become neither too lengthy nor pointed. Sometimes she should also move the little head by lifting it and should pull upon it in

[53] I.e. the thenar eminence.

[54] One would expect *kyphōsis* rather than *lordōsis*.

order to exercise the tendons and move the vertebrae, since by itself the infant is not able to move these parts.

34[103]. Having attended to this, the wet nurse should turn the newborn over and thoroughly anoint the front parts. Also, at intervals of a few days she should put drops into the eyes, but not every day, for in some cases it gives rise to eye trouble, sometimes even to ulceration of the membranous parts. She should again massage each outstretched hand [55] from the acromion down. Then lastly, she should cross them over the chest, drawing them towards the ribs and folding them around as is customary when people embrace, and at the same time extend them to a certain degree. In addition she should massage the abdomen and thorax, and again each outstretched leg, then both joined together. She should also move the kneecaps to and fro, lest they become hard to move through adhering to other parts.[56] And for the sake of comely form she should further smooth them out, applying her flat hand lengthwise while the legs are in juxtaposition. With the thumbs she should massage the eyes ⟨and⟩ shape the nose, raising it if flat, but pressing it if it is aquiline. And in a case of an aquiline nose she should not correct it at the top of the curve, but where it is prominent around the tip and should draw forward the raised alae of the nose. If the infant is male and it looks as though it has no foreskin, she should gently draw the tip of the foreskin forward or even hold it together with a strand of wool to fasten it. For if gradually stretched and continuously drawn forward it easily stretches and assumes its normal length, covers the glans and becomes accustomed to keep the natural good shape. In addi-

[55] Cf. above, footnote 51.
[56] Literally: "to the legs."

tion, she should shape the scrotum from where the thighs meet <and>, lest it be bruised, she should first put a piece of wool over the thighs and should thus lay it down.

35[104]. Following the massage, the newborn should be swathed, after being anointed with a small quantity of olive oil. For too much is cooling and does not allow the swaddling clothes to stay in place because of the moisture, and when they slip and turn, the limbs become distorted. Also it is sometimes advisable to anoint the body with Etruscan wax melted <together with> olive oil before swaddling. For this softens and warms the body and furthermore it somehow nourishes and whitens [57] it. After the bath she should aspirate the ears and nose of the newborn, lest remaining moisture harm the natural ducts which are as yet delicate.

XVII[XXXVII]. *How and When to Give the Newborn the Breast.*

36[105]. Having let a little time pass so that <the newborn may rest after> the disturbance of the bath, the wet nurse should put it to the breast. For to give the food immediately is harmful, not only for a child, but for an adult too, since the constituents of the body when warmed attract the food suddenly and spoil it. And the wet nurse herself, if she just comes from a bath, should let sufficient time pass and should first drink a little water. For it is not only harmful for an upset body to take food, but also food from an upset body is harmful. Thus the child as well as the person who

[57] According to Galen, "De compositione medicamentorum per genera" I, 12 (ed. Kühn, vol. 13, p. 411), Etruscan (literally "Tyrrhenian") wax was not naturally white.

feeds it should wait after the bath; <and> the nurse should first milk out what lies in the breasts and, having squeezed out the milk spoiled by the disturbance, she should then give pure food when the body is calm.

37[106]. Always indeed when giving the breast, the wet nurse should sit down. With her bent arms she should press the newborn against her bosom, letting it lie on its side in a slightly raised position, now on its right, now on its left side, and she should put the nipple between its lips. And she should sit with her head bent forward as if nodding, since if she bends backwards or leans forward, swallowing becomes too difficult, so that sometimes what is being drunk is returned, while sometimes it even causes suffocation. For the same reason moreover the newborn should lie in a slightly raised position; and not continuously on the right side: first, in order to change about and feed it on each breast; second, lest the right hand, if not always exercised, remain inactive after the removal of the swaddling clothes. Now, having inserted the breast as has been said, and before the child draws on the nipple, the wet nurse should gently express the milk to provoke the appetite and lest the child suffer for a long time when it strains for the first draught. If the wet nurse gets up from her sleep she should always walk about, rubbing and shaking the breasts, <and> should then offer the milk to the suckling. For the superfluous matter evaporates and the thick particles are dissolved by such previous activity. And having held the infant in her bent arms for a little while after it has partaken of the right amount of milk, she should lay it down in a bed such as we have indicated [58] so that it peeps out and bends forward, as in a little chair. Always, however, she should drape something over it from above for a cover, or

[58] Cf. book II, 16.

she should cover up the eyes themselves with some material. This should be done not only because they are easily harmed through their delicacy by anything that may fall into them, but also because through too much light and unpleasant gleam they are likely to squint. Besides, the newborn should not sleep with her, especially in the beginning, lest unawares she roll over and cause it to be bruised or suffocated. For this reason the cradle should either stand alongside the bed, or if she wants to have the newborn still nearer, the crib [59] should be placed upon the bed.

38[107]. One should advise the wet nurse not to give milk at all times during the day and night. For through such excess the newborn is overcome by disease, since it takes new milk before having digested the first, thus spoiling the first, and this is especially true at night. To be sure, one should give the breast several times since the newborn is not able to take as much food as is sufficient. For milk is by nature filling, so that it satiates the child before enough has been given for its nourishment. Besides, the newborn itself, wearied through lack of strength in drawing longer at the nipple, gives up before having taken enough. For this reason one must give it milk several times, but not incessantly, not before the bath, and far less during the bath itself, as women obstinately do who wish to silence an infant that cries easily. For if the milk becomes spoiled and sour the nervous system [60] suffers and epilepsy and apoplectic attacks take place. But worst of all is to leave the nipple in the mouth while the infant goes to sleep to prevent it from crying altogether. For when the nose is compressed, the mouth blocked, and the pharynx

[59] I.e. a trough made up as a bed; cf. above, p. 87.
[60] *Neurōdes*, cf. above, p. 93.

pressed upon, then the milk flows sometimes without sucking and the infant strangles.

39[108]. Above all, one <must> not always give the child <the> breast because it cries. First, since sometimes crying does it good. For it is a natural exercise to strengthen the breath and the respiratory organs, and by the tension of the dilated ducts the distribution of food is more readily effected. But one should not let it cry too long, for this harms the eyes and moreover causes a slipping down of the intestines into the scrotum.[61] Second, the newborn does not only cry because of hunger, but also because of an uncomfortable position from constriction or pressure, or because of the biting [62] of faeces or of some animal, or because of a sting, or a large amount of food burdening the body, or because of cold, or <heat, or> because it cannot move its bowels since too hard a faecal mass lies in the intestines, or because of some other discomfort or disease. Each of these points can be determined within limits so that one may act according to the trouble, and one should not in all cases proceed to give the newborn the breast.

Now in case the infant is bruised we shall know it by feeling with a finger the pressure from the bandage and by seeing that an extremity is becoming livid or is not in a natural position. In case it is bitten or stung by something, we shall recognize this by the fact that it has suddenly screamed although its position has not been altered nor has it been squeezed by the swaddling clothes. In case it is burdened by the offer of too much food, this will be recognized by lack of appetite and by belching, often by distention of the hypo-

[61] I.e. a scrotal hernia.

[62] Soranus often expresses our concept of "irritation" by the picture of "biting."

chondriac region (and one can determine this too from the number of times it has drunk milk).[63] In case it is chilly, this will be recognized if it becomes stiff and curls up and feels cold, sometimes also if its naked parts are livid and if the room in which it is nursed seems cold. In case it feels hot, this will be recognized if we perceive that the air is too warm, that the child is red and pants, or often if it has been covered with more covers than necessary. That the faeces are exceedingly hard and difficult to pass can be recognized from the fact that crying is accompanied by tension and spasticity of the body; that it cries <because of another> malaise or a disease of whatsoever kind: from the fact that its features are pinched and it rejects the breast without any of the above-mentioned causes. An infant will be recognized as desiring food if, when none of the indicated conditions is present, it moves its lips and opens its little mouth (especially if one touches it with a finger and by the touch reminds it of the nipple); and furthermore, by considering with how much milk the child is usually satisfied, what amount it has taken at present and whether, after a lengthy interval, <the> hypochondriac region has become flat.[64] For if the wet nurse now gives the breast to the newborn in order to restore the infant crying for want of food, she will not make a mistake.

40[109]. One must also beware of moving the child about immediately after it is satiated with milk. For adults too are harmed if exposed to shaking motions after a meal, since the food is spoiled; and much more so the child which is still young, because of the delicacy of the body and because the milk somehow tends by nature to rise. For this reason, as

[63] Caelius Aurelianus, *Gynaecia* (p. 55, 1430): "querentes quotiens aliquantum lactis acceperit."

[64] Cf. above, p. 111.

is to be expected, the newborn vomits more often when it is nauseated by an irregular and constant movement and ⟨its⟩ stomach upset in a way similar to that of people who sail and cannot stand the sea. And therefore, if children are nursed in this manner it makes their bodies moist and susceptible to disease; they suffer a thing similar to kids which are being fattened. The people who especially aim to make them fat hang them up in a round plaited basket when they have been filled with milk and move them throughout the day and night. For thus the food is carried into the whole body by the rocking movement and every part becomes distended and filled.

If, however, the newborn cries constantly after nursing, the wet nurse should hold it in her arms, and soothe its wailing by patting, babbling, and making gentle sounds, without, however, in addition frightening or disquieting it by loud noises or other threats. For fright arising from such things becomes the cause of afflictions, sometimes of the body, sometimes of the soul. One ought not then to rock the infant immediately after the meal, but either after the meal has been digested or before the meal. However, exercise in the form of rocking should be performed in proportion to the condition of the body, at first a little, by shaking the crib [65] or by suspending the cradle or by balancing it upon diagonally opposed stones. Later on the infant should be rocked in a litter; moreover, when it is four months old the wet nurse should hold it in her arms and walk about or be rocked in a carriage drawn by animals. For we do not believe in lifting it upon the shoulders and moving it about, since the testicles, if bruised, sometimes retract into the upper parts, sometimes dissolve and thus some boys become cryptorchids, others eunuchs.

[65] Cf. above, p. 110.

XVIII[XXXVIII]. *On the Dropping Off of the Umbilical Cord.*

41[110]. Now it is necessary to consider the rest of the instructions in accordance with the passage of time. First, when the umbilical cord has withered and dropped off, after three or four days, or as many as there may be, one must heal the little wound which is left at the base. Now most women burn and grind the ankle bone [66] of a pig, <or> snails or the bulbs of purse tassels,[67] and sprinkle this over while others use lead which has been heated and washed. It is still better if they mould the lead in the shape of a spinning whorl and press it upon the region of the umbilicus. Since the material is cooling, the wound will cicatrize and since it is heavy, the umbilicus will be properly moulded into a cavity.

XIX[XXXIX]. *When and How to Unswaddle the Child.*

42[111]. As time goes on one must free the child of the swaddling clothes. Now some people do this about the fortieth day, the majority about the sixtieth, while others assign a period which is even longer than this. Since in our opinion, however, the swaddling clothes serve to give firmness and an undistorted figure, we deem it right to loosen them when the body has already become reasonably firm and when there is no longer fear of any of its parts being distorted. In some cases this comes about more quickly because of a better struc-

[66] *Astragalos,* probably the talus which in pigs has a cubiform shape; cf. Joseph Hyrtl, *Onomatologia anatomica,* Wien, 1880, p. 525.

[67] Celsus, v, 2 mentions "bulbs" and "snails ground with their shells" among the drugs that agglutinate wounds.

ture of the body, while in others it comes about more slowly because of a weaker physique. But one should neither remove the swaddling clothes suddenly, nor all of them at once, for any sudden change to the opposite brings about discomfort.[68] ⟨Thus⟩ one should first free one hand, after some days the other, and then the feet. And one should liberate the right hand first. For if it is restrained according to the practice of those who free the left hand first, it becomes comparatively weak, because it gets exercise later than the other, so that also for this reason some people become left-handed. When the infant has become firmer one should also give up bathing it in its room and should take it to the bath room, but not for too long at a time nor should it be very hot. For it is not possible to give the air in the infant's room so suitable and even a temperature. If, however, the infant, while still in its swaddling clothes, is chafed by the friction of the bandages or by some other cause leading to soreness, one must give up the swaddling clothes, dress it in a simple little shirt, and heal the wounds.

XX[XL]. *How One Should Make the Infant Sit Up and Endeavor to Walk.*

43[112]. When the infant attempts to sit and to stand, one should help it in its movements. For if it is eager to sit up too early and for too long a period it usually becomes hunchbacked (the spine bending because the little body has as yet no strength). If, moreover, it is too prone to stand up and desirous of walking, the legs may become distorted in the region of the thighs.

[68] Cf. above, p. 22 and below, p. 118.

44[113]. This is observed to happen particularly in Rome; as some people assume, because cold waters flow beneath the city and the bodies are easily chilled all over; as others say, because of the frequent sexual intercourse the women have or because they have intercourse after getting drunk—but in truth it is because they do not make themselves fully acquainted with child rearing. For the women in this city do not possess sufficient devotion to look after everything as the purely Grecian women do. ⟨Now⟩ if nobody looks after the movements of the infant the limbs of the majority become distorted, as the whole weight of the body rests on the legs, while the ground is solid and hard, being paved in most cases with stones. And whenever the ground upon which the child walks is rigid, the imposed weight heavy,[69] and that which carries it tender—then of necessity the limbs give in a little, since the bones have not yet become strong.

45[114]. Therefore when the child first begins to sit up, one should support it by covering it with clothes,[70] or one should prop it up by putting things capable of holding it at its sides, but not for a long time at first. When it is making more progress so that it crawls and stands up a little, one should place it by a wall and leave it there, and later on by a chair on wheels. In this way, progressing little by little, it will practise walking. So much for its movements, and now we must also give instructions about the food.

[69] Plato, *Laws* VII; 789 E thinks that nurses should carry children until they are three years old "as a precaution against the danger of distorting their legs by overpressure while they are still young" (Bury's translation, Loeb Classical Library, vol. 2, p. 9).

[70] The meaning seems to be that some clothes be wrapped tightly around the infant's body so as to act as a corset.

XXI[XLI]. *When and How to Wean the Infant.*

46[115]. Now until the child has become firm, it should only be fed milk. For while the pores [71] are still narrow, it is not safe to proceed to more solid food. The latter moves slowly in the process of distribution because of the narrowness of the passages, yet bruises everything that is supposed to receive it. Therefore those women are too hasty who, after only forty days, try to give cereal food (as do those for the most part ⟨who⟩ find nursing a burden). Yet, on the other hand, it is also bad not to change to other food when the body has already become solid—not only because the body becomes moist and therefore delicate if fed on milk for too long a time, but also because in case of sickness the milk easily turns sour.

For this reason, when the body has already become firm and ready to receive more solid food, which it will scarcely do successfully before the age of six months, it is proper to feed the child also with cereal food: with crumbs of bread softened with hydromel or milk, sweet wine, or honey wine. Later one should also give soup made from spelt, a very moist porridge, and an egg that can be sipped. But one should beware of giving milk to drink during the meal, for the food becomes difficult to digest since it floats on top of the fluid milk; moreover, the thirst is not quenched. Sometimes, therefore, when the infant is very thirsty after the meal one should give it water or a little watery wine through artificial nipples, for out of these it draws the fluid little by little as from the breasts without being harmed. Sometimes, however, one should offer a soft

[71] Soranus here seems to accept the atomistic theory of Asclepiades by referring to the pores as internal interstices through which the food has to move when being conveyed to the various parts of the body; cf. also *Anonymus Londinensis,* ed. Jones, pp. 88–89, and Introduction, p. xxxiii.

piece of bread dipped in diluted wine, for the morsels which the wet nurse has formed by munching are harmful because of being combined with phlegm. However, one should reject bread flavored with poppy or sesame and everything spicy, for any of these is even difficult for adults to digest.

47[116]. As soon as the infant takes cereal food readily and when the growth of the teeth assures the division and trituration of more solid things (which in the majority of cases takes place around the third or fourth half-year), one must stealthily and gradually take it off the breast and wean it by adding constantly to the amount of other food but diminishing the quantity of milk. For thus the infant will be weaned without harm, getting away little by little from the first habit. At the same time the milk of the child's nurse will simply dry up because of the gradual elimination of sucking. For it is harmful to anoint the nipple with some bitter and ill-smelling things and thus wean the infant suddenly, because the sudden change has an injurious [72] effect and because sometimes the infant becomes ill when the stomach is damaged by the drugs.

48[117]. The best season for weaning is the spring, which is relatively healthy because of the well-tempered climate. For weaning in the autumn is bad, for then the whole body, on account of the unevenness of the climate, is disposed to disease, and one must avoid changes of habit which are somehow unpleasant because unaccustomed.[73] One should, however, not pay attention to Mnesitheus and Aristanax who maintain that one should wean a female six months later because it is weaker; for they do not realize that some female

[72] The Greek expression (*xenismon empoiein*) implies the harmful effect of something strange and unaccustomed; cf. the following note.

[73] The idea that sudden change to unaccustomed things has an injurious effect occurs repeatedly in this work; cf. above, pp. 22, 115.

infants are both stronger and fleshier than many males. One should not alienate the child from anything: neither from the drinking of wine, water, cold and hot things, nor from anything fatty, for it is good to create a habit for useful things straight from the beginning. Yet one should not cease nursing before teething takes place. If the infant's body is too heavy and it is short of breath it will be necessary to keep the flesh within bounds in this way: the wet nurse must have fewer and not very rich meals and must drink water; while she should give milk to the infant infrequently and should have it exercise by means of a little pushcart. If by nature the infant is gluttonous and desires more food than it can hold, one must divert its mind with entertainments and games ⟨and⟩ must divide the portions and give it pieces of dry bread and make the milk less rich. If, on the contrary, the infant could hold more food but desires less, one must tempt it by the variety of the things offered, for the novelty of the dishes stimulates the appetite. If, however, a weaned infant falls ill, one must change it back to milk, and after the disease has stopped and the little body has recovered, only then must one wean it.

XXII[XLII]. *On Teething.*

49[118]. About the seventh month teething takes place and from this arises inflammation of the gums, jaws, and tendons. As a prophylactic measure one should give the child nothing before this time that needs mastication, since the gums, if bruised all around, become very much irritated and are hard to split if they have grown callous. On the contrary, from the fifth month on one should persistently rub the gums during the bath with an anointed finger and soften them with chicken fat. And the brain of a hare acts the same way by reason of "antipathy."[74] One should also give the infant a piece of fat to hold in its hands, too big to be swallowed, so that it may suck its moisture; in this way the gums would not be softened unduly by the softness of the fat. But at the time of teething itself, and especially when the teeth have already cut through, one should no longer do this. For, in addition to the pain, the sockets will be distorted if the infant while sucking makes the fibers of the fat lie flaccid around the teeth. One should also omit butter and pungent ointments (for the inflamed parts are irritated by their biting qualities) and should moreover avoid lancing with the knife as harmful. One should apply soft and clean pieces of wool upon the neck, head, and jaws, and moisten these with warm sweet olive oil which is also dropped into the auditory canals. If the inflammation continues, one should, moreover, use poultices of the finest meal, or fenugreek or linseed and fomentations with sea sponges, especially for the gums, and should in addition anoint the latter with honey boiled down to the right degree. If sympathetic disturbances are marked one should omit the bath too and should see that the wet nurse drinks little, and then only water. She should take gruel-like food and when giving the breast she should gently force up the milk with her hand, ⟨lest⟩ the infant be injured by the sucking and suffer more violent inflammation.

[74] As the text stands, Soranus here seems to express belief in action by "antipathy." The whole sentence has been suspected and excluded by Ermerins. Ilberg retained it with reference to p. 47, 17, p. 121, 27 of his edition and Muscio I, 134. Muscio, it is true, mentions hare's brain, but without reference to "antipathy." The two passages in Soranus himself show him averse to any belief in the effects of antipathy other than purely psychological ones.

XXIII[XLIII]. *On Inflammation of the Tonsils.*

50[119]. If the tonsils are inflamed we make use of the same things and instill honey water and juice of barley. The nurses, however, poultice the throat with roasted cummin mixed with water, rub the tonsils with salt and old olive oil, and, seizing both legs with one hand, they place the child head downwards in the doorway and make the bregma touch the threshold of the house; [75] and this they do seven times. This position leads to a congestion of the little head and consequently of the tonsils too, and the rubbing in itself exacerbates inflammation and even more so on account of the pungency of the salt. Cummin, ⟨moreover, by reason of⟩ its powerful effluvia also leads to a congestion of the head.

XXIV[XLIV]. *On Thrush.*

51[120]. If thrush (which is a superficial ulcer located in the cavity of the mouth) occurs and if the crust is small, one should anoint the mouth with honey. But if the crust is larger and combined with dryness and inflammation, one should poultice with things which have loosening properties. If, however, it is combined with moisture one should use poultices having an astringent effect, like those prepared from lentils and pomegranate peel. Moreover, internally [76] one should apply to the ulcer the "*anthera* remedy," or the tender blossom of roses, or cyperus, or the fruit of tamarisk.

[75] The reading here is doubtful.
[76] I.e. inside the mouth.

When the ooze has been conquered to some extent, one should use medications for the mouth made of black mulberries and of poppyheads and of plantain, with honey, or any other astringent juice boiled with honey. Iris with honey is also helpful, or you may blow it on dry; furthermore, chopped leaves of roses, the blossom of roses, saffron, a little myrrh, oak gall, frankincense and the bark of the frankincense tree —together, or each of them singly—mixed with honey; and in addition to these honey water and the juice of a sweet pomegranate. But one should avoid wrapping hair around a finger, dipping it into olive oil or honey, and wiping off the ulcers as the nurses do, especially the Syrian ones; for when the crusts are torn off, the ill-treated ulcers are irritated.

XXV[XLV]. *On Exanthemata and Itching.*

52[121]. For itching of the body application of heat is helpful, as well as plenty of ointment made of refined [77] olive oil to which a little wax is added, so that the oil becomes thicker and remains longer on the body. As to exanthemata, blisters,[78] and such sores as form on the skin and are very moist, we avoid brine and urine because of their pungency . . . should be accepted readily.[79] Now, when the eruption is at its height it is time for the treatment. We prescribe bathing with a warm decoction of roses or lentils, and if we need a more astringent effect, with myrtle or mastich or

[77] I.e. purified by boiling.

[78] The Greek word is *phlyktaina* and, apart from the ophthalmological sense (cf. Galen, ed. Kühn, vol. 14, p. 774) can refer to blisters as well as pustules.

[79] The text is corrupt but the parallel in Paul of Aegina I, 6 suggests that skin eruptions "are to be encouraged, in the first place" (Adams' translation, vol. 1, p. 10).

bramble or pomegranate peel. We poultice more severe ulcerations with plantain and bread, or with endive, or with a powder of barley and purslane, or of houseleek or of navelwort, or with dried roses or fresh roses boiled with melilot or dates; and we use ointments of litharge, white lead, alum, vinegar, and myrtle oil, or rose oil or mastich oil.

53[122]. When the flux [80] and the great discharge of ichors have ceased and ⟨if⟩ the sores seem inflamed, we resort to bathing with a warm mixture of water and olive oil ⟨or⟩ with a decoction of linseed or fenugreek or the roots of the wild mallow, and we anoint the sores with white of egg beaten and mixed with a moist wax salve. After the disappearance of the inflammation, however, if some impurity remains we clean it away with honey boiled down moderately, so that it may lose its pungent and irritating quality, or with lentils together with honey (but it is well to boil the lentils peeled, so that they may be without their astringent husk). When the sores have become clean, we fill up the cavities to a certain degree by means of smooth litharge or white lead or "the remedy diluted with juices." [81] After the levelling, for the sake of cicatrization we apply the remedy of gum ladanum or of eggs or barleycorn or that of cadmia smeared on together with rose oil. Moreover, one should gently cleanse with natron for the child will not tolerate the stronger remedies. It is, however, very good to prescribe a rather sweet diet to the wet nurse and it is also very good to put the infant itself on a diet, not

[80] Literally: *rheumatismos*. The word used to indicate any flow of humors until Baillou in his *Liber de rheumatismo* (1642) gave it the present connotation of rheumatism.

[81] The Greek words for "with juices" are *dia chylōn*. Galen (ed. Kühn, vol. 13, pp. 831 and 996 ff.) gives the prescription of various *diachylōn* remedies in which according to the formulae of Menecrates (cf. Galen *ibid.* p. 996 ff.) litharge plays a great role. This probably accounts for the modern connotation of "diachylon."

satiating it nor, on the other hand, starving it. But if the infant's bowels do not move, one should pour out honey and boil it down to the size of a suppository; if even so the bowels do not respond, one should add turpentine to the quantity of a chick-pea. If, however, the bowels are loose, one should give millet above all.

XXVI[XLVI]. *On Wheezing and Coughing.*

54[123]. When the child wheezes because of the accumulation of much phlegm, some people prescribe lozenges of cardamom, cummin, nettle seed, and pepper. We, however, eschew these on account of their pungency, since irritating things provoke a flux and become the cause of more inflammation. Instead, we continually give drops of honey water and if the child, not yet able to spit, swallows the phlegm, we press its tongue and when thus vomiting takes place, the swallowed matter is easily evacuated. When the infant coughs, we make use of lozenges prepared with small pine cones, roasted almonds, linseed, the juice of licorice, pine seed, tragacanth, and honey—and again we avoid pungent substances (for they aggravate the cough which is as yet new) [82] and we omit the bath too.

XXVII[XLVII]. *On Siriasis (seiriasis).*

55[124]. Siriasis, as Demetrius states in his book on "Semeiotics," is nothing but a burning fever. According to some people, however, it is an inflammation of the parts

[82] I.e. "not yet chronic" (Liddell and Scott, p. 1529).

around the brain and the meninges so that as a consequence the bregma and the eyes sink in; at the same time there is paleness and dryness of the body and anorexia. When siriasis occurs one should do everything as in a case of inflammation.

Now some people ⟨say⟩ that the disease ⟨is named⟩ *seiriasis* after the star [83] because of the heat, but according to others it is called after the sunken bregma, because among farmers *seiros* is the name of a hollow object in which they throw and keep the seed.

These patients too benefit by the yolk of an egg diluted with rose oil and applied upon the bregma in the form of a pledget, and constantly changed. Or again one may put upon the bregma the leaf of heliotrope, grated pumpkin, the skin surrounding the flesh of a melon or the juice of the black nightshade together with rose oil.

XXVIII [XLVIII]. *On Flux* [84] *of the Bowels.*

56 [125]. When the infant suffers from a flux of the bowels, we omit bathing and passive exercise. Instead we apply astringent plasters, and we inject a cyath [85] of the juice of plantain or of something of this kind by means of a small ear syringe: in general, things which we likewise approve for adult patients, so long as the strength permits. If the infant takes the breast we put the wet nurse on a regimen corresponding to the affliction of the infant, ordering her to abstain from bathing, to drink water and to take astringent food, for its quality is carried upward [86] so that the child gets a

[83] I.e. Sirius, the dog star, which reigns during the dog days.

[84] Cf. above, footnote 80.

[85] I.e. "about 1/12 of a pint" (Liddell and Scott, s.v.).

[86] I.e. to the breast.

greater share of it. For just as sows which eat darnels [87] cause dizziness in the sucklings they feed, without themselves becoming dizzy, and just as kids nursed by goats eating scammony are purged [88] although the bowels of the goats do not become loose, so by eating astringent food the wet nurse is but slightly constipated, the infant, however, which is fed by her milk much more so. For this reason, in the opposite case, 〈when〉 the infant remains without a bowel movement for some time, we give the wet nurse things which loosen the bowels.

57[126]. For as a general rule, as long as the infant is nursed, we put the wet nurse on a regimen appropriate to the disease of the child, while for the child we make an appropriate use of plasters, poultices or compresses. For a weaned child, however, we prescribe food appropriate to the disease, and for these things one may refer to what we shall say about therapeutics.[89]

At what age the child should be handed over to a pedagogue and what kind of a person he should be, and in what manner the child should be prepared by him for the parents if not brought up by them, and all problems of this sort do not belong to the realm of medicine. They belong more to the realm of philosophy, so that we leave it to others to break with custom and philosophize, while we ourselves [90] here bring to an end the discourse on child rearing. Having thus com-

[87] Aristotle, "De somno et vigilia" 3; 456 b 30, mentions darnels among the hypnotics.

[88] Galen (ed. Kühn, vol. 17 B, p. 306) also tells that the milk of goats that eat the offshoots of scammony in spring acquires a cathartic quality.

[89] This reference is not clear. Possibly Soranus means that the therapeutic parts of his works *On Acute* and *Chronic Diseases* or some other of his works should be consulted.

[90] We have accepted Ermerin's conjecture of *autoi* instead of *autois* (Ilberg 93, 14).

pletely finished the discussion of things normal, we must go more deeply into the main topics which deal with things abnormal in women.[91] And that the character of the argument may be clear we shall first examine the meaning of the question whether women have conditions peculiarly their own.

[91] On the division of the book and the concepts of "normal" and "abnormal" cf. Introduction (p. xl) and p. 3.

‹ BOOK III ›

Whether Women Have Conditions Peculiarly Their Own.

1. The inquiry is also put forward in this way: whether females have conditions peculiarly their own, in as much as "woman" is a species, and "female" a genus. "Their own," moreover, is used in many ways and, with reference to the present subject, in two ways: that which does not belong to another (in this meaning one says that a garment is one's own since it is held as private property), and that which is not alien (in this meaning each of two brothers with joint property calls the estate or slave his own although it is just as much the property of the other). This inquiry refers to the first meaning. "Condition" is either said of something according to nature (like conception, childbirth, and lactation) or of something contrary to nature (like fever). Again in the case of "against nature" it is either taken in a general and generic sense (as constriction) [1] or in a particular and specific

[1] "Constriction" denotes a condition shared by many diseases according to the methodist sect, just as the term "tumor," in modern medicine, covers a great variety of growths.

sense (as phrenitis or lethargy). The discourse deals chiefly with what is contrary to nature, both in general and in particular.

2. The inquiry is useful in order to ascertain whether, moreover, women need therapy peculiarly their own. Now a disagreement has arisen. Some assume that there are special diseases of women, as do the empiricists, Diocles in his first book "On Gynecology," the Erasistrateans Athenion [2] and Miltiades, the Asclepiadeans Lucius in his third book on "Chronic Diseases," and Demetrius of Apameia. Others, however, assume that there are no special diseases of women, as for example do Erasistratus and Herophilus in the opinion of the majority, as has been noted, and Apollonius Mys in his first and third book, "<On> the Sect," and, in the opinion of the majority, Asclepiades and Alexander Philaletes, Themison and Thessalus and their followers. [3]

3. In defense of the existence of diseases peculiar to women, arguments such as the following are advanced: we call some physicians women's physicians because they treat the conditions of women. And the public is wont to call in midwives in cases of sickness when the women suffer something peculiar which they do not have in common with men. Furthermore, the female is by nature different from the male, so much so that Aristotle [4] and Zenon the Epicurean say that the female is imperfect, the male, however, perfect. Now that which is different in its whole nature will also be subject to its own diseases. Besides, the uterus is a part peculiar to women and the functions of the uterus appear in them alone, as menstrua-

[2] There is a lacuna in the text where the title of Athenion's book or the names of other physicians may have stood.

[3] I.e. the methodists.

[4] Aristotle, "De gener. animal." I, 20; 728 a 17 f. says that "it is through a certain incapacity that the female is female . . ." (*Oxford transl.*).

tion, conception, parturition . . .[5] seven primary and simple diseases; and therefore no disease peculiar to women will be amongst them.

Herophilus, moreover, in his "Midwifery" says that the uterus is woven from the same stuff as the other parts, and it is regulated by the same forces, and it has available the same substances, and that it suffers disease from the same causes (for instance: quantity, thickness, and variation of similar things).[6] Consequently there is no condition in women peculiarly their own except conception, pregnancy, parturition, lactation, and conditions antagonistic to these. The Asclepiadeans, contending that there is no condition in women peculiarly their own, say that the female is composed of the same elementary particles [7] as is the male, and is rendered ill by the same cause (i.e. obstruction,[8] for they say that this is the actual cause of most diseases) and is cured by <the> same operations and diets. Thus they say that females have no conditions peculiarly their own, since the physiology, etiology, and therapy is a general one. But Themison and Thessalus † besides those in the other parts of the body . . .[9] and for this reason they say that a condition peculiar to women does not exist.

[5] The end of the arguments for the existence of special diseases of women as well as the beginning of the arguments against their existence is missing. The enumeration of authorities above in chapter 2 indicates whose opinions may have been outlined.

[6] The meaning of this parenthesis is not clear. Possibly Herophilus by "similar things" refers to the "similar parts" of Aristotle and Galen, such as fat, nerve, and other "tissues." The meaning would then be that the uterus becomes diseased by changes in quantity, consistency, and variation of its component tissues.

[7] I.e. atoms which, according to Asclepiades, form the body.

[8] I.e. of the pores and ducts of the body.

[9] The corruption of the text (see dagger sign) and a lacuna make the passage unclear.

4. With these men we agree and ⟨maintain⟩ that the others are mistaken in their argument. For we do not say that our body is a "triple-web" [10] and that its economy depends on the substances consumed,[11] nor that the predisposing cause of disease is a plethora of the blood and the actual cause its transfusion and difficult passage.[12] Besides, it is not true that there ⟨are⟩ seven genera of diseases as we show in detail elsewhere. Furthermore, it is possible that along with the specific "weave" of the primary constituents some part may have developed in women which is different (for Erasistratus says that other parts also have become quite different through the specific combination of the vessels). And even if it is not different it may be affected differently, since the same part sometimes suffers from constriction, sometimes from flux. Similar things have also to be said against Herophilus and against Asclepiades who is wrong in his concept of the elements and about causation also. Besides, he says that obstruction [13] is not the actual cause of all, but of most diseases, because ravenous hunger, dropsy, and fever from exhaustion are produced by another cause. It is consequently possible on his thesis that a disease peculiar to women may arise without being brought about by obstruction, as happens in difficult labor.

5. In their bare statements all these men are correct, but

[10] According to Erasistratus, whose opinions are here combated, all organs consist of a triple web of arteries, veins, and nerves in between which the *parenchyma* is poured.

[11] I.e. food and pneuma; cf. *Anonymous Londinensis* XXII, 50 (ed. Jones, p. 86).

[12] Erasistratus believed that normally the arteries contained pneuma and the veins blood. If, however, blood filled the veins to excess, a plethora would result and the blood would also enter the arteries and obstruct the course of the pneuma.

[13] Cf. above, p. 130.

in their arguments they are wrong. Now we say that there exist natural conditions in women peculiarly their own (as conception, parturition, and lactation if one wishes to call these functions conditions [14]), whereas conditions contrary to nature are not generically different but only in a specific and particular way. For in regard to generic differences, the female has her illness in common with the male, she suffers from constriction or from flux, either acutely or chronically, and she is subject to the same seasonal differences, to gradations of disease, to lack of strength, and to the different foreign bodies, sores, and injuries. Only as far as particulars [15] and specific variations are concerned does the female show conditions peculiarly her own, i.e. a different character of symptoms. Therefore she is subject to treatment generically the same, as will be understood more plainly by the following remarks.

I. *On the Retention of the Menstrual Flux and on Difficult and Painful Menstruation.*

6. Of the ailments to be treated by diet [16] we deal first with the retention of the menstrual flux, since menstruation is the first function of the uterus. However, painful and difficult menstruation is different from retention (just as obstructed and difficult urination is different from retention of the urine). Retention is an absolute damming of the blood which flows naturally through the uterus, whereas difficult menstru-

[14] The Greek term, *pathos,* implies suffering, i.e. a pathological condition.
[15] This could also be translated by "localization."
[16] Cf. Introduction, p. xi. Surgical disorders are discussed in book IV.

ation is an impediment of its discharge. Moreover, not to menstruate is also different from having the menstrual flux retained. For while retention means absence of menstruation, absence of menstruation does not necessarily mean retention of the menstrual flux, e.g. in women who are too young and too old and in certain other similar cases. For here it is absurd to talk of retention of the menses, where there is nothing to be menstruated. Hence not to menstruate is the more general principle and common to physiological and pathological states, whereas retention of the menstrual flux is subordinate and always pathological.

7. Now of those who do not menstruate, some have no ailment and it is physiological for them not to menstruate: either because of their age (as in those too young or on the contrary too old) or because they are pregnant, or mannish, or barren singers and athletes in whom nothing is left over for menstruation, everything being consumed by the exercises or changed into tissue. Others, however, do not menstruate because of a disease of the uterus, or of the rest of the body, or of both: "of the uterus" if <the> condition of so-called imperforation is present, or callosity, or scirrhus, or inflammation, or if a scar has formed on a sore, or a closure of the orifice (from long widowhood among other causes), or a flexure; "of the rest of the body," e.g. when it is subject to undernourishment, great emaciation and wasting, or to the accumulation of fatty flesh, or cachexia, or fevers and long ailment, or if through hemorrhoids, vomiting, or nasal hemorrhage, the substance [17] is taken instead to these parts.

8. During the interview one must, therefore, note the patient's age and this is found out by inquiring after the

[17] I.e. the material that physiologically would be used for the menses.

number of her years; we recognize pregnancy from what we pointed out above,[18] and mannish women from their appearance, and habits and manner of life by questioning. We recognize those who do not menstruate on account of an ailment of the uterus by the healthy state of the rest of the body, and those where the condition is caused by an ailment in the region of the female organs, or in the rest of the body, by the fact that menstruation which formerly was manifest is no longer present while the woman is still in her bloom; further by the fact that heaviness of the loins or tension or pain in the pubic region and the groins is present; or that the stomach is upset and sluggish and that there is singing in the ears and impediment of sight, or heaviness or pain in the head, or burning of the face; that the vessels around the back of the head bulge, and that the roots of the eyes ache. When, however, there is at the same time lack of menstruation from one of the physiological causes (e.g. if pregnancy is present and one of the conditions which usually check the menstrual flux), we discover from the additional signs that the retention has not come about by reason of the disease. If, however, this escapes us there is no harm done, since we do not do anything specific about the retention of the menses, but remove the whole underlying disease directly, whether it checks the menstrual flux or not.

9. Now one should not treat those without disease for whom it is physiological not to menstruate because of their age. For they are not troubled in any way and besides, to change nature is either impossible or not easy and sometimes even dangerous. For if the pathological state is the opposite of the physiological, the physiological if changed into its opposite necessarily becomes pathological. Nor should one

[18] Cf. book I, 44; above, p. 43.

treat those who do not menstruate because of gymnastic training or vigorous vocal exercise, inasmuch as they have no disease. If, however, they seek to menstruate because they do not conceive, one must make them live more genteelly by restricting their active mode of life so that their bodies may become more feminine. But those who do not menstruate because of some ailment must be treated according to the disease that has caused the retention of the menstrual flux. One should cut away the hymen or tissue for those in whom there is no perforation,[19] soften and alter the consistency of the callosity and of the scirrhus, reduce the inflammation by gentle means, make the scar as thin as possible, relieve closures and flexures, strengthen those women who are emaciated and undernourished and make them put on flesh, change cachexia and reduce fat, prescribe baths for those who have a fever, put an end to every ailment either recent or chronic, remove hemorrhoids, check vomiting and hemorrhage from the nose. To some extent we have indicated the particular treatment for every single one of these in our other works on therapeutics; and we shall expound upon it in part here. In any case, even if the menstrual flux is retained through an ailment in another part of the body, it is advisable to treat the uterus locally too by means of massage and remedies which have a hardening effect, as we shall point out a little later.

10. As a general rule, when a constricted state [20] develops in the region of the uterus, the menstrual flow is sometimes retained completely, sometimes it becomes difficult and painful; now colic is present and pains in the groins, loins, and pubic region, now in the head, the tendons of the neck, the

[19] Cf. above, p. 133.

[20] This refers to the basic condition of *status strictus* as assumed by the methodist school; cf. Introduction, p. xxxii.

eyes, the hips and thighs; the breasts are swollen, appetite is lacking, the genitals are hot and dry—all of which, in the woman so disposed, occurs about the time of menstruation. We shall now state the treatment of this condition.

When the pains set in or when the menstrual flux is entirely retained, one should put the woman to bed in a room which is moderately warm and bright and should see that she is quiet but awake and fasts completely; and one should lightly press her extremities and those parts that suffer excessive pain. For it is not only by the innate heat that each of the constricted parts is relaxed, rather the throbbing of the pain is assuaged by the resistance of the pressure too. If, however, the pain does not yield, one should also apply warm fomentations: either warm cloths, or linen towels and wool, and warming pans filled with warm water, or bladders containing warm olive oil, or ground grain, lukewarm, in bags, or a sea sponge wrung out in boiling water and wrapped up in a cloth so that the parts may not be cooled by the moisture but gently soothed by the influence of the vapor. Afterwards a soft clean piece of wool soaked and wrung out in warm sweet olive oil should be applied to the pubes and abdomen and at the same time to the loins and hips; moreover one should continue to keep these parts moist with oil increasingly warm; while warm water is to be given as a mouthwash and for drinking.

But if the initial stage [21] is less severe one should allow the woman to sleep. One should also use poultices of linseed or of bread kneaded in warm hydromel, and sitz baths as they will be described later,[22] and at the beginning of the first three-

[21] *Epitasis;* cf. Introduction, p. xxxv.
[22] Cf. the following article.

day period [23] one should give a rub down with an ointment, give a mouthwash and warm and simple food.

11. If, however, the pains are very vehement, then before or on the third day one should let blood from the bend of the arm opposite to the more <painful parts>, because withdrawing blood from the less affected parts is less troublesome. If all parts suffer equally, one should let blood from the left arm in order to keep the right arm free for service. Venesection from the ankle, however, should be avoided as long as the vessels of the arms are visible and no inflammation is manifest around them; for the stasis [24] troubles the patient and the vessels at the ankle bones are less wide.

After the disturbance resulting from the venesection has subsided, one should rub the body and put the patient into a sitz bath prepared from warm oil mixed with water or from a decoction of fenugreek, linseed, or mallow cultivated or even wild. The labia having been separated, one should pour in the same oil together with an egg, alone or with one of the decoctions mentioned, beaten up to the thickness of glue. One should next apply to the genitals a piece of soft wool soaked in the same fluids and should then put a piece of felt around. When the disturbance has subsided, one should give warm water for a mouthwash and as a drink in order to assuage the thirst and to facilitate the digestion of food. After the drink

[23] For the methodist's treatment by three-day periods, cf. Introduction, p. xxxvi.

[24] The original reading of the manuscript has here been adopted. Rose and Ilberg changed *stasis* to *spasis* assuming the latter term to stand for *antispasis* (*revulsio*), whereby Galen (ed. Kühn, vol. 10, p. 315) meant bleeding from a vein distant from the affected organ. The history of this concept has been treated in detail by John B. de C. M. Saunders and Charles Donald O'Malley in *Andreas Vesalius Bruxellensis: The Bloodletting Letter of 1539*, New York, Schuman, 1947.

one should give a little simple light food, warm and in the form of a gruel, e.g. spelt prepared with water or with honey water boiled down moderately; or the spelt gruel made with honey or olive oil, dill, and a little salt; or bread soaked in water or else together with eggs that can be sipped. After a short interval following the meal one should allow the patient to sleep. Afterwards, until the illness is on its decline, one should keep the patient on a restricted diet and should give food every second day, provided that the strength of the body does not fail. ⟨On the third day after venesection⟩ [25] one should employ cupping, dry at first and not only during the remissions but during the attacks as well, in order to diminish the pain; it should be applied gently without causing too much pulling (for it is possible to prevent an excessive degree of suction if a spatulate probe is inserted along some part of the lip of the thin cupping vessel). Later, however, cupping may also be combined with superficial scarification and should be performed on the pubes and the hypochondriac region when the ailment is at its height but the initial stage abating.[26] But when the condition lasts one should use leeches too, a piece of linen being first laid under them that they may not cause a chill. The leeches draw blood more actively if the area has first been swollen by a cupping vessel and a dressing of lint has been applied, lest the animals be hindered from fastening upon the lacerations by the greasiness of the other parts. After the leeches have fallen off and if but little blood has been drawn, one should apply cupping vessels where it seems necessary; otherwise one should cover the bites with small pieces of lint and should spread over them a piece of

[25] The text has a lacuna here, the bracketed words being supplied from Muscio's version; cf. Ilberg, apparatus.

[26] Cf. Introduction, p. xxxv.

linen soaked in oil, then a piece of wool. Afterwards one should use poultices which have a relaxing effect, e.g. bread kneaded with fresh warm pork fat or with boiled and well-ground wild mallow roots; or linseed with the finest meal or with fenugreek; or all three boiled together with olive oil, honey, and the decoction of mallow or fenugreek. One should, however, change the first poultices constantly, for if they stay on they cool and become sour through the heat of the inflammation. Moreover, they should not be put on either too thin, for thus they cool quickly and dry easily, or too thick, for thus they burden the inflamed parts. Besides, one should also use an injection into the anus of warm olive oil to the amount of four cyaths, and simple suppositories.[27]

12. For the ancients were wrong in prescribing so-called blood-drawing suppositories for bringing the blood down, and draughts producing the same result. They did not realize that the draughts harm and upset the stomach, while corroding suppositories ulcerate the uterus and thus produce deep ulcerations of an evil character which heal poorly, while over the ulcerations a scar forms which is thicker than any normal flesh, so that the menstrual catharsis may be retained. And in general all such draughts and suppositories, being of pungent power, act as irritants upon inflammation and thus double the pains and enhance the impediment to menstruation. For just as it is not good to use pungent collyria when the eyes are inflamed, nor irritating remedies in dysuria or difficult defecation, by the same token one should not use pungent things when the uterus is inflamed in very painful menstruation. For such are the remedies which among the ancients had a reputation for bringing blood: e.g. squirting cucumber, black hellebore, pellitory, panax balm, drugs which women

[27] Cf. below, ch. 13.

have often used also for abortion.[28] As I have just said, everything pungent and irritating should be avoided; instead one should choose that which is likely to relax gently.

13. The best suppository is a piece of wool soaked in warm, sweet olive oil. One may also beat juice of fenugreek or linseed or mallow with oil into a thick mass and boil any of these with fresh goose or chicken fat, so that one can separate the fatty cream and spread it on a piece of wool. Also: yolk of egg triturated with these and perhaps reduced into one mass by means of refined honey. Also: a decoction of melilot in sweet wine. Or: the inner part of juicy dates similarly boiled with sweet wine, the skin having been removed because it is slightly astringent. One should also apply heat externally by means of sea sponges wrung out in hot water or oil mixed with water, or a decoction of fenugreek, linseed, or mallow, either cultivated or wild. However, the sponges should be changed constantly and a piece of linen put beneath them and the parts abundantly anointed with warm olive oil so that the area may not be chilled.

14. When the treatment has progressed well, then one should advise swinging in a hammock. When the acute stage has passed the menstrual flow appears forthwith; nevertheless, after it has ended one should prescribe restorative treatment: bathing, varied food, and wine, as well as rocking, promenading, active exercises, and massage of the whole body as well as of the region around the uterus. However, in the local massage of the uterus strokes with the bare hands cause bruising; therefore, when the patient sits down in a good-sized bowl to be washed <or> when she steps down to the bathing tub, one should put flat and soft sea sponges round

[28] Cf. book I, 64; above p. 66, where Soranus himself prescribes panax balm for abortion.

the lower abdomen and the hips and, gently pressing with the hands, one should move them to and fro ⟨and⟩ should gradually increase the amount of massage. One should also advise cerates with marjoram oil, or oil of lilies, or some similar oil and should not only instil them but should also smear them all over the orifice and neck of the uterus; moreover, one should employ suppositories of relatively high emollient power, such as the one prepared with wax, turpentine, ox fat with enough sweet olive or henna oil to make all the rest of the ingredients of thick consistency; also the suppository prepared of juices [29] and any one made of marrow, fat, and relaxing seeds. The so-called marjoram remedy for the relief of pain also belongs here. A bath of olive oil is also very useful.

15. If, however, the condition has become chronic one should apply the same treatment during the attacks. But in the intervals one should first apply the restorative cure,[30] the materials needed for which we have mentioned and here one should also employ the services of an experienced anointer. Second, one should make use of the metasyncritic cure.[31] The latter must be preceded by a day of complete fasting, but if the patient cannot endure this, one must keep her on water and limited food. Then it is necessary to divide the loaf of bread into portions of such size as may be most easily digested. One must divide it into two parts: one half should be cut into three equal portions, while the other half should be given together with a little preserved meat or fish and pungent additional dishes for two, three, or four days,[32]

[29] Cf. book II, 53; above, p. 123.

[30] Cf. above, article 14.

[31] The metasyncritic cure was of major importance in the treatment of chronic diseases by the methodist school; cf. Introduction, p. xxxv.

[32] This is the period of "pungent diet."

starting on the day after the fast. Then one should switch to bland foods like vegetables, delicate fish, and brain; next, for an equal length of time one should change <to> fowl, and for an equal number of days <to> fresh pork. And with every change from one diet to the other, one should also take one of the three portions of the half loaf; furthermore, on the first day of each change, one should omit wine and the bath, but should have both on the next day.

Except for the period of pungent diet alone, one should advise local remedies also, namely on the day following the transition from one diet to another. Sometimes one should use cupping for metasyncritic purposes, sometimes apply intense heat, sometimes a pitch plaster on the pubic region and the loins, and a sprinkling of natron, salt, and irritating lotions, sometimes fomentation, sitz baths in sea water, and a rubefacient of mustard, and shower baths. If, however, the affliction is not cured, one must no longer start out with fasting alone, but must in addition provoke vomiting with radishes.

16. One should also use irritating cataplasms like the one with bayberries or that with seeds, and suppositories producing the same effect, and their use is opportune after the ending of menstruation. For when the time of menstruation is near one must omit drastic and disturbing remedies. Particularly, for such suppositories one should use rue ground with honey, or the so-called "thin-leaved" fleabane, or raisins without stones ground with natron or salt; furthermore, cummin, pepper, absinthium, hyssop, butter, old olive oil, and similar things. These should be smeared into a suppository the size of a bean, dipped into sweet olive oil or oil of lilies to take the edge off the sting, and placed before the orifice of the womb. With the same substances one should

anoint the groins too, and should lubricate the anus internally. For just as stubborn diseases of the eye sometimes terminate in the eyelids becoming hard and rough and therefore requiring pungent and metasyncritic collyria for the complete removal of the disease, so the parts around the uterus too sometimes remain hard ⟨and⟩ rough and callous, so to say, when the inflammation has abated a little, and need a certain sharp stimulant for their metasyncrisis. If, ⟨however,⟩ even so the condition is unrelieved, one must make the patient choke with white hellebore and must afterwards prescribe prolonged traveling, the use of natural waters, and, in general, diversion of the mind. For if by thus keeping on with the same things and adding more active ones the condition is relieved, menstruation becomes unimpeded.

II. *On Inflammation of the Uterus.*

17. "Inflammation" (*phlegmonē*) derives its name from "inflame" (*phlegein*) and not, as Democritus said, from phlegm (*phlegma*) being its cause. There are many conditions which precede the inflammation of the uterus, but the more frequent are cold, likewise pain, miscarriage,[33] and a badly managed delivery, none of which makes any difference in the treatment.[34] When the uterus is inflamed some general signs appear and some particular ones, the latter indicating what part of it is affected. For sometimes the whole womb is inflamed, othertimes its orifice, neck, the fundus, or cavity,

[33] For definition of the term (*ektrōsis*) cf. below, p. 170.

[34] This is another example of the indifference of the methodist sect to etiological research. According to Soranus it is the condition itself, i.e. inflammation of the uterus, that is of therapeutic significance, whereas it does not matter what caused it.

either above, below, or on the sides, and sometimes several of these, or the majority of them.

The general signs which appear are the following: fever, furthermore pain and pulsation of the affected part, swelling and <rigidity>, heat and dryness of the abdomen, tense feeling in the hips or heaviness in the loins, flanks, lower abdomen, groins, and thighs, spells of shivering, a stabbing sensation, numbness of the feet and coldness of the knees, profuse perspiration, a small and very rapid pulse, sympathetic affection of the stomach, fainting, and weakness; during the initial stage,[35] moreover, hiccups, pains in the throat, jaws, bregma, and eyes, particularly in the back of the eyes, hindrance of urine, faeces, or even of both. If the inflammation becomes worse, fever and swelling of the abdomen increase, delirium sets in as well as gnashing of the teeth <and> convulsions.

18. These are the general signs, while the particular signs, when the orifice alone is inflamed, are: closure of the orifice accompanied by a painful feeling; the orifice inclines toward the anus, and the groins especially and the genital region are tense. If the orifice is not inflamed as a whole, but in part, the same areas show partial tension; there appears furthermore, a swelling which is painful <to> the touch and a deviation in the direction opposite to the swelling. For if the right side is inflamed the orifice deviates toward the left; if, however, the left, toward the right; if its lower part is inflamed it points more upward, but if the upper part is inflamed it is more inclined toward the anus than in any other case.

19. One has to consider whether the pain is on the same side as the inflammation, or whether by spreading it has taken hold of the opposite parts too. Among our predecessors

[35] *Epitasis;* cf. Introduction, p. xxxv.

some say that the opposite groin and thigh ache, whereas Demetrius the Apamean maintains that the pain is located on the side directly involved. For he thinks that it is not plausible that the area near the inflamed part should not be painful, while pain should be felt in the parts which are not affected (as some people have believed who concentrated only on the passing of the inflammatory process to the opposite parts and its attacking that area). For in his opinion it is more logical that these parts too become sensitive only after the immediate surroundings of the inflamed part have undergone much tension, and because the process passes on to the opposite side. We agree on this point, even though this argument does not make any difference as to the use of local treatment.

20. If the neck is inflamed the sympathetic reactions are greater and the swelling lies behind the orifice. And if the right part is inflamed the leg on the same side is affected and the groin swollen; and if the left, then things are reversed. If the lower part, which lies upon the beginning of the rectum, is inflamed, there is difficulty in passing faeces,[36] retention of faeces, and urgency as in tenesmus; giving a clyster is not easy, and if one inserts the finger into the anus one encounters a swelling which seems to be around the rectum. If, however, the upper part is inflamed there is dysuria <and> the pain is more in the pubic region and pudenda. But if the whole neck is inflamed all the aforesaid signs are present and because of the increased swelling the cervix bulges into the vagina.

21. If the cavity of the uterus is inflamed at the sides, pain

[36] The reading of the Paris Ms. (*dysōdia* instead of *dysodia* as corrected by the editors) would mean: "the faeces have a foul smell." This, as Drabkin noted, must also have been the reading of the Greek text at Caelius Aurelianus' disposal since the latter translates (*Gynaecia*, p. 73, 294): "sequitur teter odor viscerum."

develops in <the> corresponding flank and becomes more violent when the patient turns upon the opposite side. But if the inflammation is in the anterior and upper parts there is more pain and swelling in the abdomen, dysuria, or retention of urine; and after urination the swelling is more easily felt. If the inflammation has its seat in the posterior and lower parts of the cavity there is more pain in the loins and it is aggravated when the patient bends forward or to the side; the clyster is not easily given, the faeces are retained, flatus is not passed, and the finger introduced into the anus <meets> with a swelling <which seems to be around the rectum. However, this can be differentiated> from inflammation of the rectum by the fact that pain does not immediately set in when the finger presses, but follows when the pressure lasts for some time; furthermore by the fact that the swelling is displaced so that the bowel regains its proper position; and by the fact that the swelling shifts when the woman changes to a kneeling posture; none of which happens when the rectum is inflamed.<If the fundus is inflamed, pain,> tension, and heaviness are felt alongside the umbilicus toward the loin; [37] often, moreover, the orifice is retracted and drawn inward when the parts above the neck are inflamed, so that some say that the uterus is not affected.

22. If the whole uterus is inflamed all signs are present together; the sympathetic reactions are severe and there is a greater swelling of the abdomen. From an inflammation developing in the abdominal wall we differentiate this condition by the fact that in it the swelling or the redness does not show so much externally, nor does the swelling remain

[37] This (literal) translation of the Greek text is hard to understand. Caelius Aurelianus (*Gynaecia,* p. 73, 319) says more clearly: "secundum umbilicum atque clunes."

fixed whatever the posture, but moves about, while the skin follows the pull of the fingers. Whereas, if the abdominal wall is inflamed, the opposite of this takes place and the pain is more external, while urination is unhindered. Likewise we differentiate between inflammation of the uterus and peritoneum by the fact that in the latter the swelling is not circumscribed and the urine is either not hindered at all, or not in proportion to the swelling. As a rule, in inflammations of the uterus the head and neck are sympathetically affected, while in inflammation of the abdomen and the peritoneum they are little affected or not at all.

23. This then is the differential diagnosis, but now we shall turn to the therapy. One should follow the same recommendations we have mentioned above in connection with painful menstruation. In the beginning we make the patient lie down in a bright and moderately warm room, prescribing rest and a complete fast. We rub and hold the legs and wrists; we apply warm fomentations, which we keep moist and cover with clean pieces of wool; giving an instillation we evacuate the bowels by means of a relaxing clyster, i.e. warm sweet olive oil and the like. One should give warm water for a drink and mouthwash and warm, gruel-like food . . . afterwards gently relaxing poultices, cupping, and scarification; one should put leeches on or give a sitz bath or hot sponge bath, an injection of warm olive oil by means of a clyster, a simple suppository . . . and give suppositories of a relatively high emollient power, a bath, and varied food, later also tart and thin watery wine.

24. If in addition fever develops, one should not change the treatment. Rather, one should see to it that something is done during the paroxysms, while during the remissions one should bring about a change in the predisposing cause with-

out altering the treatment. Themison is therefore deserving of censure when, in the third book of "Chronic Diseases," he approves of relaxing remedies in inflammation without fever, while in inflammation with fever he advises astringent remedies, the juice of black nightshade and *perdikion.* He is deceived by the concomitant heat [38] into prescribing cooling remedies and later even rose oil in water, without realizing that things which increase inflammation also heighten the heat. Indeed, according to Themison himself, one must assuage the symptoms with things which do not aggravate the disease. Likewise one should avoid all those pungent suppositories which some of the ancients used, oil with an infusion of rue and greasy wool, butter and bread with rose oil, parsley oil and a mixture of oil and vinegar. For everything pungent and acrid irritates inflammation and makes it more violent.

III. *On Satyriasis.*

25. Satyriasis occurs more often in men and therefore we have dealt with it at length in the work "On Acute Diseases"; [39] but it also occurs in women. They show intense itching of the genitals together with pain, so that they continually bring their hands to this region. Because of this they develop an irresistible desire for sexual intercourse and a certain alienation of mind (because of the sympathetic relation of the meninges with the uterus) which throws aside all sense of shame. . . .

[38] I.e. of the fever.

[39] Caelius Aurelianus, *Acute Dis.* III, ch. 18.

IV. *On Hysterical Suffocation.*

26. Hysterical suffocation (*hysterikē pnix*) has been named after both the affected organ and one symptom, viz. suffocation (*pnix*). But its connotation is: obstructed respiration together with aphonia and a seizure of the senses caused by some condition of the uterus. In most cases the disease is preceded by recurrent miscarriages,[40] premature birth, long widowhood, retention of menses and the end of ordinary childbearing or inflation of the uterus. When an attack occurs, sufferers from the disease collapse, show aphonia, labored breathing, a seizure of the senses, clenching of the teeth, stridor, convulsive contraction of the extremities (but sometimes only weakness), upper abdominal distention, retraction of the uterus, swelling of the thorax, bulging of the network of vessels of the face. The whole body is cool, covered with perspiration, the pulse stops or is very small. In the majority of cases they recover quickly from the collapse and usually recall what has happened; head and tendons ache and sometimes they are even deranged.

27. The hysterical disease, on account of the aphonia and seizure of the senses, is related to epilepsy, apoplexy, catalepsy, lethargy, and the aphonia caused by worms.[41] All these taken together as a unity may be differentiated by the fact that in these diseases the uterus is found to be normal or not much affected, while in the hysterical disease it is greatly inflamed and retracted. Moreover, while hysterical women,

[40] For definition of the term (*ektrōsis*) cf. below, p. 170.

[41] All these diseases are discussed at length by Caelius Aurelianus in his Latin paraphrase of Soranus' works on acute and chronic diseases.

in the majority of cases, recall what they have suffered once the paroxysm is over, this is not the case with women who suffer from the other diseases. Hysterical women have had much trouble with the uterus, while of the others those who are aphonic because of worms have trouble with the intestines and abdomen, and the rest have headaches. Epileptic women, moreover, show froth and a big pulse; not so hysterical women.[42] In apoplectic patients the pulse is strong, whereas in hysterical patients it is weak. The latter are distinguished from cataleptic patients by the fact that catalepsy is connected with fever; [43] the eyelids are wide open and the teeth clenched before the height of the fever, but relaxed at its height —while hysterical suffocation is without fever and the eyelids are shut. To lethargic patients it is peculiar that they become comatose during fever [43] and have a big pulse—which is not the case in hysterical women. And to those who suffer from aphonia because of worms it is peculiar to cry out from time to time and to have an uneven and intermittent pulse.

28. This then is the differentiation of hysterical from related conditions. ⟨The disease⟩ is of the constricted and violent class and exists both in an acute and chronic form; therefore the treatment must be suitable to these characteristics. During the initial stage [44] one should lay the patient down in a room which is moderately warm and bright and, without hurting her, rouse her from the collapsed state by moving the jaw, placing warm compresses all over the middle of her body, gently straightening out all the cramped

[42] Cf. Owsei Temkin, *The Falling Sickness,* Baltimore, Johns Hopkins Press, 1945, p. 50.

[43] Catalepsy as well as lethargy are here considered as febrile diseases and, therefore, not identical with the modern definitions of these terms.

[44] *Epitasis;* cf. Introduction, p. xxxv.

parts, restraining each extremity, and warming all the cool parts by the touch of <the> bare hands. Then one should wash the face with a sponge soaked in warm water, for sponging the face has a vitalizing effect.

If, however, the state of aphonia persists, we also use dry cupping over the groin, pubes, and the neighboring regions; then we put on covers of soft clean wool. We also moisten these parts freely with sweet olive oil, keeping it up for some time, and swathe each extremity in wool (for this conducts the relaxation from the extremities toward the center). Then we instill warm water into the opened jaws, and afterwards honey water too, and prescribe movement in a hammock. When the initial stage [45] has ended we bleed, provided that weakness does not prevent it, or it is not long since food was given. Afterwards we give an injection of warm, sweet olive oil, moisten the parts, offer warm water as a mouthwash and drink, and make her abstain from food until the third day. On this day we first rub the patient down and afterwards we offer gruel-like food and give this from now on, every second day, until the dangerous condition regarding the uterus has safely subsided. <But every day> we use poultices like those prescribed for women who suffer from painful menstruation [46] and apply hot sponge baths and relaxing sitz baths, the material for which we have mentioned above,[47] and suppositories made of fat, marrow, fenugreek, mallow, and oil of lilies or henna oil, and injections by means of a clyster of olive oil or oil mixed with water, particularly if faeces are retained (for the excrement bruises the adjacent uterus). When the

[45] *Epitasis;* cf. Introduction, p. xxxv.
[46] Cf. above, pp. 136, 139.
[47] Cf. above, p. 137.

condition has abated we make use of wax salves and suppositories of a relatively high emollient power, then we give varied food, later on a bath, and finally wine.

If paroxysms and remissions occur frequently and if, therefore, the disease is chronic, one should use the abovementioned things during the paroxysm; whereas during the interval one should first restore the patient by various passive exercises and promenades, reading aloud, vocal exercise, anointing, gymnastics, baths, and varied food. Then one should effect a metasyncrisis by means of a pungent diet, a pitch plaster, cupping, intense heat, vigorous local massage, sprinkling powders, sitz baths containing pungent ingredients, irritating suppositories <and> cataplasms, mustard plasters and the "cyclic treatment." [48] If, however, the condition does not clear up, then one must also make the patient choke by means of white hellebore after having provoked vomiting by means of radishes, order traveling on land and sea, and prescribe natural waters. We have described the proper use of all these things in our work "On Therapeutics."

29. But the majority of the ancients and almost all followers of the other sects have made use of ill-smelling odors (such as burnt hair, extinguished lamp wicks, charred deer's horn, burnt wool, burnt flock, skins, and rags, castoreum with which they anoint the nose and ears, pitch, cedar resin, bitumen, squashed bed bugs, and all substances which are supposed to have an oppressive smell) in the opinion that the uterus flees from evil smells. Wherefore they have also fumigated with fragrant substances from below, and have approved of suppositories of spikenard <and> storax, so that the uterus fleeing the first-mentioned odors, but pursuing the last-mentioned, might move from the upper to the lower parts.

[48] Cf. above, article 15.

Besides, Hippocrates made some of his patients drink a decoction of cabbage,[49] others asses' [50] milk; and he, believing that the uterus is twisted like the intestines are in intestinal obstruction, inserted a small pipe and blew air into the vagina by means of a blacksmith's bellows, thus causing dilatation.[51] Diocles, however, in the third book "On Gynecology," pinches the nostrils, but opens the mouth and applies a sternutative; moreover, with the hand he pushes the uterus toward the lower parts by pressing upon the hypochondriac region; and applies warm fomentations to the legs. Mantias gives castoreum and bitumen in wine to drink and if the arousal is imminent, he orders playing on the flute and drumming. Xenophon proposes torchlight and prescribes the making of greater noise by whetting and beating metal plates. And Asclepiades applies a sternutative, constricts the hypochondriac region with bandages and strings of gut, shouts loudly, blows vinegar into the nose, allows sexual intercourse during remissions, drinking of water ⟨and pouring cold water over the head.⟩ We, however, censure all these men who start by hurting the inflamed parts and cause torpor by the effluvia of ill-smelling substances. For the uterus does not issue forth like a wild animal from the lair, delighted by fragrant odors and fleeing bad odors; rather it is drawn together because of the stricture caused by the inflammation. Also upsetting the stomach, which suffers from sympathetic inflammation, with toxic and pungent potions makes trouble. Forcing air by means of the smith's bellows into the vagina—this

[49] Cf. Hippocrates, "On Women's Diseases" II, 123 (ed. Littré, vol. 8, p. 266).

[50] Cf. Hippocrates, "On the Nature of Women," ch. 3 (ed. Littré, vol. 7, p. 314 f.), and "On Women's Diseases" II, 131 (ed. Littré, vol. 8, p. 278).

[51] Cf. Hippocrates, "On the Nature of Women," ch. 14 (ed. Littré, vol. 7, p. 332), where, however, blacksmith's bellows are not mentioned.

inflation makes the uterus even more tense, which is already rendered sufficiently tense by reason of the inflammation. Moreover, the use of sternutatives, through their shaking effects and the pungency of the drugs, produces a metasyncrisis in chronic conditions, thus aggravating the condition of the patient who during the initial stage [52] needs not force but gentleness. Sounds and the noise of metal plates have an overpowering effect and irritate those who are made sensitive by inflammation. At any rate, even many healthy persons have been given headaches by such sounds. Vinegar blown in is also harmful, for just as external inflammations, so internal inflammations are increased by every astringent. Furthermore, it is injurious to constrict externally with strings or bandages the inflamed uterus which cannot even bear a poultice without feeling it burdensome, because of the intensification caused by the pressure. And drinking of water is not ⟨only⟩ not helpful but sometimes even noxious, since the patient needs strengthening, not metasyncrisis; moreover, ⟨metasyncrisis⟩ is produced again by switching to diluted wine. Intercourse causes atony in everybody and is therefore not appropriate; for without giving any advantage it affects the body adversely by making it atonic. Pouring cold water over the head in order to stop aphonia is obviously a technical mistake. For if the body is rendered dense by the cold, the arousal necessarily becomes more difficult to accomplish on account of the increased inflammation.

v. ⟨*On Tension of the Uterus.*⟩

30. . . .

[52] ***Epitasis;*** **cf. Introduction, p. xxxv.**

VI. *On Air in the Uterus.*

31. Air in the uterus occurs after expulsion of the fetus, from cold, abortion, or difficult labor when the orifice is closed or blocked by a clot, similar to the other . . . and sometimes it [53] is pushing toward the right groin, sometimes toward the left. Moreover, the psoas muscles [54] and the hips are also painful in some patients, and signs of a sympathetic reaction with the uterus, such as pains in the tendons, headaches, etc., are observed. And there is slight pitting on pressure with the fingers, quickly replaced, however, by swelling. Furthermore, upon tapping with the hand a tympanitic note is observed; sometimes also colic, and a stabbing sensation which runs through like the pulse. Relief is induced by warmth, then follows an exacerbation, noises, and rumblings as if one felt outside air running through. The semen introduced during intercourse is destroyed. Symptoms of the swelling are constant in some cases, while in others they occur at certain intervals.

32. Now one must arrange the plan of treatment as for a state of constriction,[55] with relaxing injections and poultices, dry cupping and cupping with scarification, and all remedies of a similar kind. The patients should not take food which is difficult to digest and take care of and which is pungent or causes flatulence; rather they should take food that can be easily taken care of. The midwife, having first anointed her finger, should insert it and remove the embedded clot if it

[53] The beginning of the symptomatology is missing and it is impossible to say what the "it" refers to.

[54] *Psoai;* Galen's (ed. Kühn, vol. 18 B, p. 100) description of the psoas muscles agrees approximately with their modern description.

[55] I.e. *status strictus.*

lies within reach, touching it gently to loosen it, so that the discharge may be unimpeded. And if air in the uterus becomes a chronic condition we use more relaxing remedies during exacerbations (for in attacks and exacerbations we recommend similar things). But when a remission takes place, we strengthen the body by means of warm ointments and by general and topical massage of the legs and the affected parts, performed sometimes with the bare hands, sometimes with very rough dry linen; and we give varied, sometimes even pungent, food. The loins and the abdomen we anoint by means of a pitch plaster and besprinkle them with natron or apply intense heat; we also use a rubefacient of mustard and dried figs, or poultice with barley together with boiled figs, rue, hyssop, and honey. We also apply the plaster made of natron, figs, and absinthium, or ground grain with boiled figs and hyssop, or "the seed cataplasm," or that of Polyarchus, or that with bayberry; the latter we at first use along with a wax salve, then alone. We also employ similar substances in preparing sitz baths, boiling carrots, Cretan daucus, and pennyroyal in water and, if the condition persists, wormwood, hyssop, horehound, sweet bay or its fruit, cassia, and spikenard. In addition we use suppositories of the same character, namely of rue, ⟨pennyroyal⟩, honey, natron, and turpentine: mixed with galbanum, iris, rue, hyssop, and ox bile in equal or unequal parts. Of the same class is the following suppository:

Of rich figs ground so that the seeds do not show	1 drachm
⟨Very soft root of cyclamen	2 drachms
White aphronitre	1 drachm⟩

And in order to weaken its great pungency and sting, it is advisable first to dip the suppository in milk and insert it.

Also one should apply to the affected parts cupping vessels in a circular pattern and should detach them forcibly; sometimes one should even use them combined with scarification. And one should make use of everything that is apt to cause metasyncrisis, such as natural waters, shower baths and swimming, the temperature warm at first, later on cold; thus gradually accustoming the body to stand the cold so that the affected parts may be strengthened. Food should be given which makes one thin and which is apt to dissolve the gases.[56] Furthermore, one should use the Diospolis remedy and sometimes also the "mint remedy."

33. However, we omit the more drastic remedies because the stomach becomes upset; also burning of scents, and fumigating with aromatic substances. For when the head becomes congested by them it suffers harm which is greater than the benefit. Likewise we reject astringent plasters, e.g. those made with quinces, Theban dates, tart wine, bloom of the wild vine, acacia, or pomegranate peel. For air in the uterus, having developed from a state of constriction, is not dispelled by astringent remedies but by loosening and relaxing ones.

VII. *On Soft Swelling of the Uterus.*

34. When the uterus shows soft swelling a yellowish, spongy, soft tumor develops which yields upon pressure of the fingers and comes out again shortly afterwards. The surface of the abdomen is of the same color and rises up if pulled with the fingers. Now one has to use the same reme-

[56] The use of the term "gas" is anachronistic since it was introduced by Van Helmont in the 17th century only. Soranus has *pneumata* whereby he means the air-like substances in the uterus and intestines.

dies as we have mentioned for air in the uterus. And one should irrigate the affected parts first with warm olive oil, later on with henna oil or oil of iris; moreover ⟨one should use⟩ suppositories similar ⟨to those used for⟩ air in the uterus.

VIII. *On Scirrhus and Sclerotic Changes in the Uterus.*

35. Partial or total hardening of the uterus develops after inflammation. A hard resistant tumor appears which upon forceful pressure induces a feeling of numbness. And just as in sciatica the patients, in walking about and stooping, have a pain in the loins, the groins, the abdomen. . . .

IX. *On the Mole* (mylē).

36. The so-called *mylē*—or *mylos* as others say—is a hardening of the uterus which arises because of a preceding inflammation, sometimes also because of a localized ulcer that has developed an excess of flesh. It has been named *mylos* [57] from its immobility and heaviness. Sometimes it develops in a part of the uterus, e.g. the orifice and the neck, so that the tumor meets the inserted fingers, the whole mass pressing downward. But in the majority of cases it develops in the

[57] Literally: "millstone." According to Galen (ed. Kühn, vol. 10, p. 987) *mylē* is the name for unformed flesh. Hippocrates, "On Women's Diseases" I, 71 (ed. Littré, vol. 8, p. 148 f.) gives the following account of the etiology of a mole: "This is the cause of a mole in pregnancy. If the women in whom the menses are abundant conceive little and sickly seed, no proper fetus develops; the abdomen is full as of a pregnant woman yet nothing moves within the abdomen, nor is milk formed in the breasts although they become plump." Oribasius (*Collect. med.* 22, 6; vol. 3, p. 65) likewise connects mole with pregnancy. As Lüneburg (p. 119, note), however, rightly remarked, Soranus' description might fit a number of conditions.

whole uterus and is then attended by a hard, stone-like tumor which is manifest in the abdominal region; at the same time the hypochondriac region, which lies higher up, is drawn down [58] and there is emaciation, paleness, and anorexia.

37. At first it has the appearance of a pregnancy: the menses stop, the breasts swell, the stomach is upset while the loins ache, and the abdomen swells. But as time goes on it is differentiated by the occurrence of stabbing pains but without any movement as in the pregnant. Later, when the whole body wastes and when the swelling increases it takes on the appearance of dropsy. It is, however, differentiated from dropsy by the fact that upon pressure with the hand the swelling never yields nor becomes pitted, and upon tapping with the hand no tympanitic note or wave obtains, as in dropsy. Occasionally, when in the course of time the liver cools down, dropsy develops in addition. Some say that in a few patients a dense piece of flesh about the size of a nut grows through the vagina, in some patients in the course of a month, in others in the course of two or three months.[59]

38. Some have given up the above disease as incurable, others have treated incipient cases only, whereas we treat it even after it has become chronic. And one should not be negligent; indeed, during exacerbations—which we recognize from the increased heaviness and feeling of numbness, or the poor digestion of food, and insomnia occurring without any manifest cause—one should treat with warm relaxing poul-

[58] This probably means a flattening out of the contents of the hypochondrium.

[59] Caelius Aurelianus (*Gynaecia,* p. 82, 529) interprets differently "nunc per singulos menses, nunc interpositis duobus vel tribus." Although his translation agrees well with the Greek text it is difficult to interpret medically. Soranus' emphasis, in the following paragraph, on the treatment of the chronic disease is characteristic of the attention to chronic conditions given by Themison and the methodist school.

tices, cupping, scarification, leeches, heat, soothing relaxing injections, softening suppositories, sitz baths, cerates boiled with marsh mallow and sweet olive oil or henna oil, the diachylon [60] cataplasm or that of Mnaseas; one should give food which produces good humors and has good juices, and should provide a lift toward the shoulders by means of a bandage, in order to alleviate the distress that has been caused by the pull downward. Now these are the things one should do during exacerbations. In addition, during remissions we strengthen the whole body by means of the restorative cure,[61] passive exercises, promenades, baths, vocal exercises, a little wine, and suitable and varied foods. And we change the condition of the parts first affected by means of a pitch plaster, application of intense heat, sun baths, sprinkling of natron and salt, and massage. Furthermore, we use a rubefacient of mustard and dried figs and cataplasms, that with seeds as well as that with bayberries, and Polyarchus' cataplasm and that of Cephisophon, and similar ones; moreover, such sitz baths and hot applications as may cause metasyncrisis (e.g. <with> boiled sea water or brine, with a decoction of sweet bay, bayberry, pennyroyal, hyssop, salvia, horehound, wormwood, dittany, centaury, germander, garlic germander), and vaginal suppositories made with butter, hyssop, goose fat, chicken fat, deer's marrow or brain and honey, or the flesh of dried rich figs and raisins together with old olive oil, or henna oil, or oil of iris, or marjoram, or *amarakos*, or lilies, or *malabathron*. If the condition progresses one should also try a pungent diet, the cyclic cure,[62] the use of natural waters and shower baths

[60] See book II, 53; above, p. 123.
[61] See above, articles 14 and 15.
[62] See Introduction, p. xxxv.

and swimming in the sea or in natural waters, and should try to provoke vomiting with radishes and—if the strength of the patient allows—with hellebore too.

39. One should beware of too pungent vaginal suppositories and sitz baths of the same type, lest by their continuous use we inadvertently irritate the scirrhous parts and besides give the disease an evil character. We reject fumigations with saffron, storax, resin, and myrrh, steaming with wormwood, pennyroyal, and the leaves of horehound and garlic germander, and the drinking of honey wine ⟨in⟩ a decoction of nosesmart and pennyroyal, for the above-mentioned reasons.[63] In most cases the treatment previously recommended has brought about a sudden discharge of a large amount of clotted and blackened blood by which the disease has been removed.

x. *On Hemorrhage of the Uterus.*

40. Hemorrhage of the uterus occurs as a result of difficult labor, or miscarriage,[64] or erosion by ulceration, or a porous condition, or from the bursting of blood vessels from whatever cause. It is clearly recognized from the sudden and excessive rush of blood, and, besides, the patients become weak, shrunken, thin, pale, and if the condition persists, suffer from anorexia.[65] Sometimes, however, it also seems to come on periodically. It is a grievous calamity, for it is impossible to treat it by pressure with the fingers, insertion of hooks,[66]

[63] Cf. above p. 157.
[64] For definition of the term (*ektrōsis*) cf. below, p. 170.
[65] This picture corresponds to chronic anemia in cancer.
[66] Hooks with which the blood vessels were twisted were used as hemostats.

plugging with pledgets, constriction with ligatures,[67] or by stitching. The blood flows not only from the uterus but from the vagina too, and some people in diagnosing the seat say that the blood flowing from the vagina is thin, yellowish, and warm, while that from the uterus is thicker, darker, and colder. But one can determine the affected part more safely by using a speculum.

41. Yet, as for treatment, the following is proper. The woman should lie down in a relatively small, dark, and moderately cool room upon a hard bed that does not move and is raised a little at the foot. She should have rest and should remain in one position (for all movement provokes a flux), and the thighs should be brought together and crossed (for this position simulates the action of a press). Clean, soft, flat sea sponges soaked in cold water, or vinegar diluted with water, or vinegar alone should be applied to the genitals, the pubes, the hips and the loins, and later on to the chest too, and should frequently be renewed. And the extremities should be gripped tightly and bandaged (for the compression resulting from this squeezing is transmitted all the way to the affected part). The face should either be dipped in cold water or sponged with pure water and fanned from time to time; and the head should be moistened with cold, freshly made olive oil and the patient should have a drink of vinegar. She <should take> sitz baths of cold water up to the groin, or of diluted vinegar, or pure vinegar, or a decoction of myrtle berries, or dried roses, or "*omphakitis* oak gall," or myrtle and lentils, or mastich, or pomegranate peel, or bramble blossoms, or leaves of oak or of willow, or tanning sumach.

However, if upon getting up the malady becomes more

[67] This is another instance showing that ligatures to stop bleeding were known in antiquity.

troublesome, the juice of any one of the things mentioned or the juice of plantain or knotgrass or endive or black nightshade or fleawort or *perdikion* should be injected by means of small clyster pipes or a uterine syringe. And if the hemorrhage persists, the juice of hypocist and acacia, as well as opium (mixed with vinegar either all together or singly), or *omphakion*, to the amount of two cyaths, should also be used. And a soft piece of wool soaked in any one of the said juices should be inserted into the orifice of the uterus with a finger or a probe, particularly if the hemorrhage comes from there. For if the hemorrhage comes from the parts above, the wedged-in piece of wool hinders the flux, but retains the discharged blood in the cavity. In such a case a soft clean sea sponge which is small and oblong and soaked with the same substances should be inserted as far inside as possible, so that the discharged blood may be absorbed and may not clot and thus cause sympathetic reactions and inflammations. From time to time one should change the sponge. It is also good to apply cupping vessels with much heat to the loins, groins, and flanks (and if possible to the hips also), to let them stay attached as long as necessary, and then take them off gently. On the same places to which we applied sea sponges [68] one should use plasters made of dates soaked in tart wine or in vinegar, together with a cerate of roses or of quinces, or with ground leaves of myrtle or medlars, or with alum, or aloe, or bloom of the wild vine, or hypocist, or acacia, or with "*omphakitis* oak gall" and freshly made olive oil, or oil of roses, or myrtle, or mastich, or quinces. Or again we use plasters made with some astringent and cooling herb (like purslane, henbane, plantain, fleawort, black nightshade, *perdikion*, knotgrass, endive) together with barley powder

[68] Cf. above, p. 162.

and vinegar or dates. And all these plasters should be changed frequently.

One should use relatively drastic vaginal suppositories, for instance oak gall, pulverized frankincense, chalcites in equal parts, together with sweet wine; or ashes of either a sea sponge soaked in raw pitch and then put inside . . . ,[69] or of the dry dregs of wine together with any of the astringent juices. If, besides, there is an erosion, one should also use the "black remedy" made of papyrus, together with vinegar, or any of the troches which are prescribed for dysentery.[70] For even if an eschar is caused by these remedies, its treatment is easy if the patient holds on to life. One should also give food after first sponging the face with cold water; and the food should consist of rice prepared in cold water or diluted vinegar, or spelt or bread and a soft boiled egg in vinegar. Then after some days she should also have endive or plantain in vinegar and a little freshly ground sumach; and after oil from freshly ground olives has been well boiled she should have this too; and apples and baked quinces or boiled pears, and a bit of meat from the breast of a ringdove boiled in diluted vinegar or stuffed with myrtle berries, or of a partridge or a francolin or anything similar to these. If the time for sympathetic reactions has passed, one should also give a little wine, and when the patient has become completely firm, a bath too.

42. However, we reject bloodletting which others as well as Themison have adopted in order to divert [71] the sanguine-

[69] Ilberg suggests that the missing words may have read "a vessel and burnt to cinder."

[70] Galen (ed. Kühn, vol. 13, pp. 86, 290 ff., 302 ff.) mentions a large number of troches, for dysentery and other diseases, from various authors.

[71] This refers to the theory current from antiquity to the Renaissance that bleeding may divert a flux; cf. also above, p. 137.

ous material. For bloodletting relaxes, <whereas> hemorrhage demands condensation and contraction; and one should not divert the material,[72] but stop it. Moreover, bleeding is dangerous because if the flow of blood is not checked by the venesection the patient necessarily succumbs more quickly, being exhausted by a double hemorrhage, as it were. If, on the other hand, it is checked with the result that later on inflammation ensues as if from an increase of irritation, there is corresponding danger. For if we were now to bleed after venesection and hemorrhage we should quickly kill the woman. On the other hand, if we did not remove blood by venesection in case of great inflammation, we should leave the patient helpless, for nothing else dispels the danger of inflammation as does bloodletting.

Some people say that some things are effective by antipathy, such as the magnet and the Assian stone and hare's rennet and certain other amulets to which we on our own part pay no attention. Yet one should not forbid their use; for even if the amulet has no direct effect, still through hope it will possibly make the patient more cheerful.

XI. *On the Flux of Women.*

43. According to the ancients, as Alexander Philalethes says in the first book "On Gynecology," the flux is "an increased flow of blood through the uterus over a protracted period." But according to Demetrius the Herophilean, it is "a flow of fluid matter through the uterus over a protracted period" since the flux may not be sanguineous only, but differ-

[72] I.e. the blood.

ent at different times. In our opinion, however, it is a chronic rheum [73] of the uterus where the secreted fluid is perceptibly increased. According to Asclepiades and some others there are two different kinds of flux (for one kind is red, the other is watery and white), whereas according to Demetrius the differences lie in color and action. In color: for one kind is white resembling barley juice, another watery, another red, another black, another slightly bloody and similar to washed meat, another is of uneven color and another is pale. In action: one kind of flux is inactive and causes neither irritation nor pain, whereas the other kind causes irritation and erosion and brings on a painful sensation at the time of its discharge. He also says that one kind comes from the whole body, another from the uterus, and a third from some other part; and they discuss these differences together with their symptomatology. It is tedious as well as useless to set forth these differences, for in every flux one must treat the whole body and the uterus locally. And the white flux is said to be more stubborn than the red, since it has to pass through narrower ducts.

As a general rule, however, we shall diagnose the flux from the fact that the genital parts are continually moistened by fluids of different color, and that the patient is pale, wastes away, lacks appetite, often becomes breathless when walking, and has swollen feet.

44. As to particulars, the disease varies as follows: One kind of flux is without pain, another with pain; and <one kind> is without ulceration, while another with ulceration which may be <either> inflamed, or dirty, or clean.

<Now if the flux is unattended by ulceration or pain, all the remedies mentioned in hemorrhage of the uterus should be

[73] Cf. above, p. 123, footnote 80.

used.> And if one wishes <to use> potions too, not toxic and pungent but mild <and astringent, one should not advise against them>. Such potions are: an infusion of sawdust from the lotus tree, either alone or with two obols of Samian earth in two cyaths of water (and if opportunity allows with tart wine too) ; or, together with it, the rennet of hare, calf, lamb, or deer (for this has a coagulating faculty) ; or ground grapestones, or myrtle berries, or pomegranate peel, or pine bark or something similar, sprinkled upon the potion to the amount of two drachms; or a decoction of Theban dates or quinces and apples.

But if the flux is attended by pain, one should inject the juice of *tragos*, spelt, or barley by means of a uterine syringe <or> a small clyster pipe. Moreover, one should apply poultices which have a warming effect and should give warm, thin food. And if the flux is accompanied by ulceration, and if the latter is inflamed, one should again use the same things as in a flux with great pain and without ulceration. If, however, the ulceration is dirty, so that the discharge looks like the dregs of wine, or if the ulceration is <clean>, one should use, just as in dysentery,[74] in some cases things that have a cleansing effect, in others such as may produce a scar. We shall mention them a little later when we discuss ulcers in the uterus.[75]

If, however, having become chronic, the flux exhibits exacerbations as well as remissions, one should use simple remedies during the exacerbations in order to give some relief. During the remissions, however, one should use things capable

[74] The analogy with dysentery may be due to the widespread assumption that dysentery was accompanied by ulcers of the intestines. See Aretaeus (Adams' translation) p. 353; Galen, ed. Kühn, vols. 7, p. 247 and 8, p. 381. Caelius Aurelianus, *Chronic Dis.* IV, 84, defines dysentery: "est autem intestinorum reumatismus cum ulceratione."

[75] This refers to book IV, ch. VI which, however, is not preserved.

of giving strength and effecting metasyncrisis; for instance, various passive exercises, promenades, vocal exercise, the restorative cure,[76] baths, wine in moderation, varied foods, intense heat, sun baths, metasyncritic cupping, pitch plasters, massage with the bare hands or with a linen towel, depilatories or metasyncritic unguents, mustard plasters, radishes to effect vomiting, a pungent diet and the cyclic cure, swimming,[77] shower baths in natural waters, a change of air by land and sea travel, sitz baths and vaginal suppositories which have an irritating action. But here too [78] we reject venesection [79] in sanguineous flux, unless violent pain demands it; for the disease needs contraction, not relaxation which the removal of blood by its very nature effects.

XII. *On the Flux of Semen.*[80]

45. The flux of semen occurs not only in men, but in women too. It is a discharge of seed without desire or erection [81] and happens at short intervals, so that the body be-

[76] "The restorative cure" rests on a conjectural emendation; the Cod. Parisinus has *aleiptikē,* i.e. "anointing," a reading supported by Caelius Aurelianus, *Gynaecia,* p. 89, 711, who has *unctionem.*

[77] Swimming in various kinds of water was discussed at Soranus' time as evinces from Oribasius' (*Collect. med.* 6, 27 and 10, 39; vols. 1, p. 523 and 2, p. 466) excerpts from Antyllus and Herodotus.

[78] I.e. as in hemorrhage of the uterus, cf. above, p. 164.

[79] Here the Cod. Parisinus added: "from the bend of the elbow, or the nose or the forehead, as we said above." Ilberg bracketed this part as an addition of the compiler. However, Caelius Aurelianus (*Gynaecia,* p. 89, 720) reads: "sive ex brachio sive ex naribus aut fronte faciendam."

[80] Literally: "gonorrhea." Th. Puschmann, *Alexander von Tralles,* vol. 1, p. 273, has pointed out that the ancient concept of "gonorrhea" covered spermatorrhea, masturbation, and gonorrhea.

[81] Literally: "tension"; Caelius Aurelianus, *Acute Dis.* III, 178: ". . . gonorrhoea, quam nos seminis lapsum vocamus, siquidem sine tensione veretri sit seminis involuntaria atque iugis elapsio."

comes pale, loses strength, and is consumed. For the uterus is relaxed, hence weakness follows, and gradually the whole body is consumed. For little by little the substance of the body flows into the uterus, undergoing a slight change in the morbid organ, as do the tears of people suffering from ophthalmia. The disease usually is chronic and belongs to the "lax" kind.[82]

46. Therefore if the disease happens to be of recent origin, one must proceed gently, just as in exacerbations. One should seat the patients in decoctions which are astringent and cool (e.g. of roses, myrtle, mastich, bramble, and similar things), and one should rub in acacia and hypocist in tart wine, and similar things, all over the lower abdomen and groins, and one should use poultices as well as cerates made of dates, quinces, and myrtle. One should place a flat, thin leaden plate beneath the loins at nighttime; the women should use a threadbare coat for a cover and the bed should not be soft.[83] Vomiting should be practised after meals, or better yet on an empty stomach. And the upper parts should be exercised and rubbed a long time, whereas the affected parts should be neither greased nor heated. One should give as a potion one drachm of the root of *halikakabon*, dried in the shade, together with water; or the seed of the chaste tree in like manner, or the seed of hemp or rue. One should not give food that has been dissolved, or which is like gruel, or engenders semen, or is irritating. Instead, the patient should mainly eat dry things and should partake of some roast fowl and a little dry wine. One should also avoid all other sexual stimulants; thus one should not show her paintings of shapely

[82] This refers to the *status laxus* on which see the Introduction, p. xxxii.

[83] This corresponds to the treatment for nocturnal pollutions as recommended by Caelius Aurelianus, *Chronic Dis.* v, ch. 7. The leaden plates are also mentioned by Galen, ed. Kühn, vols. 6, p. 446 and 12, p. 232.

forms nor tell erotic stories; rather, her diversions should be somber, and reading and narratives likewise.

If the condition becomes chronic, one should also prescribe gymnastics and make her perspire, give massage and cold baths, and continually anoint the lower abdomen and the loins with rose oil. If a remission occurs, <one must give> tonics and metasyncritic remedies, both locally and over the whole body; in regard to the requirements for this one should choose from what has been said before.[84]

XIII. *On Atony of the Uterus.*

47. Like the other parts of the body, the uterus too sometimes becomes atonic. Patients suffering from this show aversion to sexual intercourse, passing of wind, excess of black and watery menses which appear irregularly twice or three times a month, and inability to retain the seed. For in some cases the seed is shed immediately after intercourse, in others a little later after some days, in yet others after it has taken shape, and in others dead or entirely atrophied and before the term. Hence sometimes there is an "efflux," [85] sometimes "miscarriage," [86] and sometimes "premature birth." Now "efflux" is a spitting forth of the seed after the first, second, <or third> day following intercourse. "Miscarriage" is death of the fetus after the second or third month. "Premature birth" is a birth close to the completion of the fetus but before the proper time; the fetuses that have not died are

[84] Cf. book III, 15, 28 (end), 32, 38, and especially 44 (above, p. 168).

[85] Aristotle, "De gener. animal." 758 b 6, states that an abortion is called "efflux" (*ekrysis*) if it occurs at a time when the embryo resembles an egg, the fluid content being surrounded by a fine membrane.

[86] *Ektrōsis;* cf. pp. 46, 53, 143, 149, 161.

atrophic and very weak. At the time of menstruation the patients experience heaviness in the abdomen, loins, and legs. The stomach functions badly, sometimes giving rise to vapors around the head, and the same symptoms follow as in hysterical suffocation, moreover patients are sometimes seized by melancholic madness and mania. The disease results from frequent pregnancies, tensions,[87] and particularly from fetuses which are large.

48. For the treatment one should choose from the previously mentioned remedies [88] those capable of giving tone and strength to the affected parts. For one must treat this condition as a chronic lax disease.[89] During the exacerbations we ⟨also⟩ use astringent remedies, but tonics and metasyncritic remedies during the remissions. If the seed is not ejected immediately, one should assist conception as we have shown in the beginning.[90] If, however, death of the fetus is threatened, in accordance with what we indicated in a previous chapter (and when, as Hippocrates says, the breasts shrink unexpectedly, and the thighs, as Diocles notes, turn cold),[91] or even if the fetus is in process of separation,[92] one should try to prevent its expulsion. One should order much rest and should put the woman to bed slightly raised, and should apply sea sponges squeezed in diluted vinegar on her pubes and loins. For in this way miscarriage has often been mastered by the use of such treatment in recent separation.[93] But if the

[87] I.e. "tension of the uterus" to which Soranus had devoted a special chapter (ch. v), now lost.

[88] Cf. above, footnote 84.

[89] I.e. a disease of the *status laxus*.

[90] Cf. book I, 46.

[91] Cf. book I, 59.

[92] The conjectured reading of *diĕrēmenou* instead of *diephtharmenou* (cf. Ilberg, p. 126, line 17 and apparatus) has here been followed.

[93] I.e. of the fetus from the uterus.

embryo is dead, one must assist its complete expulsion by means of relaxing agents.

To go back,[94] one should use astringent sitz baths, which, however, should be lukewarm to the touch; in addition one should inject lukewarm oil of roses or narcissus or lilies or quinces into the uterus, and with similar substances anoint the hypogastric region and the loins. Besides, one should recommend that the whole body be exercised continually, using exercises suitable for a woman. Little food should be given and that mainly meat and mildly astringent. Likewise one should give moderately dry, astringent wine. The amount of fluids drunk ought to be small, for thirst is beneficial in this disease. Everything prepared with milk and cheese should be avoided and as well any purgation and looseness of the bowels.

XIV. *On Paralysis of the Uterus.*

49. The uterus is paralyzed among other causes by frequent miscarriages. Those suffering from this condition show aversion to sexual intercourse, the orifice of the uterus is cold and extremely atrophied, loosened, as if worn out, and the neck of the uterus is relaxed and anesthetic. Further, there is sometimes complete retention of the menses; sometimes they are discharged irregularly; walking is impeded as if some foreign body were lying inside, and there is an inability to conceive, since the seed during intercourse is either not placed into the uterus at all, or returns immediately as if from an inanimate vessel. Sometimes also, through sympathetic affection of the adjacent organs, an involuntary discharge of

[94] I.e. to the treatment of atony of the uterus.

urine or faeces takes place and heaviness is felt in the rectum. It is a "constricted" [95] and long-protracted disease, and has sometimes exacerbations, sometimes a remission. We shall recognize the exacerbation by the heaviness, disturbed sensibility, and increased flux; [96] the remission by the opposite. For the treatment one must choose from the remedies which have been mentioned in the chapter on retention of the menstrual flux and on difficult and painful menstruation.[97]

XV. *On Flexion, Bending, and Ascent of the Uterus.*

50. Similar to fingers that have become ankylosed, the orifice of the uterus and its neck suffer bending and flexion, sometimes laterally, forward, or backward and sometimes upward or downward, and sometimes entirely dislocated. These conditions become manifest upon insertion of the fingers (for the direction in which the distortion has taken place is perceived by touch) and through the accompanying signs. For with lateral flexion, tension, pain, and numbness arise in the corresponding leg, sometimes also atrophy, coldness, and hindrance to walking or even standing. Flexion forward and upward gives rise to hindrance of urination and to distention of the pubic region and, in some cases, even to an inability to stand. With flexion backward and downward, excretion of faeces or flatus is impeded and there is some difficulty in sitting, even more so if the flexion is toward the anus. All these are symptoms of constriction; for in cases of underlying inflammation or sclerosis or some localized stricture constriction

[95] I.e. it belongs to the class of the *status strictus*.
[96] "Increased flux" does not agree with the picture of the condition.
[97] Cf. book III, 9 ff.

is certainly present. Now some <say that inflammation> is also the cause of already existing flexion.[98] But in our opinion here again one should be guided by the condition, whether there is inflammation or, from a more general point of view, constriction. During exacerbations one ought to forbid everything pungent and irritating; instead one should use things which have a mild and relaxing effect.[99] During remissions one should employ restorative remedies and, if the disease is becoming chronic, metasyncritic remedies as well; in regard to their requirements and proper use one should refer to what has been said previously.

XVI. <*On Sterility and Barrenness.*> [100]

[98] In this place, Caelius Aurelianus (*Gynaecia,* p. 92, 785–89) is more detailed: "In lateral flexion some people have corrected the uterus with the finger placed into the anus, and have thus inserted triturated castoreum wrapped up in wool, or bitumen or liquid pitch. Then, on the next day they have adhibited rose oil and fumigations with fragrant substances mixed with water. Oblique flexion they correct with the finger and use mollifying suppositories; while in flexion forward they employ diuretic potions with bandaging of the precordia added."

[99] This follows Rose's text (p. 347, 16–17) which seems supported by Caelius Aurelianus (*Gynaecia,* p. 92, 794): "mitigativis et laxativis medemur."

[100] This chapter is preserved in Caelius Aurelianus (*Gynaecia,* ch. 64) whose version, although longer, in substance agrees with Muscio II, XVI (51).

‹ BOOK IV ›

1[XVII]. *On Difficult Labor.*

What is difficult labor?

1[53]. The Herophileans and especially Demetrius say that difficult labor is a birth that is difficult to manage; but according to some, difficult labor is a delivery attended by obstacles. . . .

What are the causes of difficult labor, and in how many ways does difficult labor occur in those who give birth in a way which is contrary to nature?

Diocles the Carystean in the second book "On Gynecology" says that primiparae and young women have difficult labor, whereas those who have often borne have easy labor. A cause of difficult labor is that the orifice of the uterus is not straight, or has become hardened and closed, and does not easily give way; furthermore he says that large fetuses are a cause too. But in the third book "On Gynecology" he says that atrophic and dead fetuses are a cause, and adds that women who are very moist and warm have difficult labor. However, he makes a mistake if he does not look for the causes which make women deliver easily; and is it not ridiculous to say that difficult labor takes place†[1] Cleophantus, however, who in the first book "On Gynecology" says that primiparae have difficult labor, adds: "and those women who are broad in the region below the shoulders but not very heavy below the hips [2] have difficult labor." "In them," he says, "the *hydrōps* <bursts> before the pangs of childbirth spread over the whole body," <and> difficult labor occurs (one must note that he calls the membrane covering the fetus *hydrōps*).[3] Moreover, he says those women have difficult labor in whom the fetus does not present by the head but by the feet, or is doubled up upon the hips or side, or has the head near the groins and one hand or one leg <thrown> forward; [4] also those women who <are> high-strung, <or> who live luxuriously or idly. For idleness is a cause of difficult labor, while exercise makes for easy labor and well-being of the fetus. But he too makes a mistake if he does not describe all the causes.

But Herophilus in his "Midwifery" says: "difficult labor at any rate occurs <because of the number> [5] for, according to Simon the Magnesian, it has repeatedly been observed that a woman has three times brought forth five children with difficulty.[6] And difficult labor takes place when the fetus is

[1] The rest of the sentence is corrupt and not understandable.

[2] This might mean a narrow pelvis as a mechanical obstacle to delivery, an interpretation which is rejected by Fasbender, *Geschichte,* p. 25.

[3] Cleophantus here ascribes difficult labor to premature rupture of membranes. On the term *hydrōps* cf. Aristotle, "Hist. animal." VII, 9; 587 a 6 where, however, it seems to denote the fluid. Soranus, on the other hand, uses the term *prorrēgma* (literally "that which burst first") and which in book I, 57 has been defined as a synonym for chorion.

[4] For a discussion of the various positions see Introduction, p. xlii.

[5] I.e. of fetuses. The reading is very uncertain.

[6] Aristotle, "Hist. animal." VII, 4; 584 b 33–36: "The largest number ever

born from an oblique position, or when the isthmus of the uterus, or also the orifice, is not sufficiently opened, or when the membrane surrounding the fetus, where the water collects, is too thick and not capable of bursting before the birth." He says that fetuses have been seen to issue forth without the membrane bursting, but that these too are born with difficulty. Difficult labor in his opinion also ⟨occurs⟩ because the uterus, or the orifice, is atonic. And atony of the uterus is a difficulty inherent in the body. "Moreover, difficult labor takes place because of external influences, diet, activities, and because of an excessive amount of bloody fluid excreted from the body. Furthermore difficulty of delivery is caused by a distention of the uterus by the fetus during the pains of labor, as well as from coldness, heat, or a growth in the abdomen or abscess in the intestines. A hollowness of the loin and spine [7] also becomes a cause of difficult labor; moreover, difficult labor occurs if there is an accumulation of fat in the abdomen and the hips so that the uterus is squeezed as it were; besides, if the fetus is dead." And this is what Herophilus said. Andreas in his work "To Sobius" (which is in the form of a letter) agrees with Herophilus' views, adding only the paralyzed and emaciated fetus: "for these," he says, "make labor difficult since they are not heavy." [8]

2[54]. But the Herophilean, Demetrius, disputes what

---

brought forth is five, and such an occurrence has been witnessed on several occasions. There was once upon a time a certain woman who had twenty children at four births; each time she had five, and most of them grew up" (*Oxford transl.*).

[7] The picture suggested is that of a lordosis. As Fasbender, *Geschichte*, p. 23, has pointed out, this is the first definite reference to a skeletal anomaly as a factor in dystocia.

[8] This apparently implies the view that the weight of the child is an active factor in childbirth.

has been said, stating that the causes of difficult labor are partly to be found in the parturient herself, partly in the child itself, and partly in the birth passage. Now difficult labor is occasioned by the parturient, when the cause is <either> in the psychic faculty or in the vital faculty, that is to say in the body. And it lies <in> the psychic faculty, when there is grief, joy, fear, timidity, lack of energy, anger <or> extreme indulgence, (for some women are spoiled and do not exert themselves). Moreover, it occurs because of ignorance of childbearing, <so that they do not> co-operate with the pains of labor. Furthermore, it happens when reason is suspended, or at least when pain is dimmed: (this one may say in the case of apoplectic and lethargic [9] women). Difficult labor also occurs because of the idea of not being pregnant.

As to the vital faculty in the body, the causes are the following: indigestion, anorexia, atrophy, dyspnoea, and hysterical suffocation. If the cause lies in <this> faculty, <he says,> [10] the condition of difficult labor is brought about when the body is very relaxed, for it cannot respond because of its lack of tonus. Or when there is much fleshiness labor will be difficult, for the ducts are narrowed; also because of excessive dissipation of the fluids in bodies which are slender. Difficult labor might also occur because the ducts [11] are narrow and the fluids retained; for the bodies which by nature are weighed down by the fluids lose their tone and, being compressed, narrow the ducts through which birth takes place. Pungent fluids or, contrariwise, mild ones which do not stimulate the body, and thick fluids likewise, cause difficult labor, the first through carrying <too much> pneuma, the others too little. Tall women

[9] Lethargy, as pointed out above, p. 150 was considered a febrile disease accompanied by a comatose state.

[10] I.e. Demetrius the Herophilean.

[11] This may refer to the pores of the body and possibly the blood vessels.

have difficult labor as also have those who are broad in the upper parts but narrow in the lower parts; [12] for they do not possess normal body proportions. In addition difficult labor occurs if the body of the uterus is afflicted by disease, e.g. if it is overheated or inflamed, or enfeebled, or paralyzed, or convulsed, or numbed. He terms these somatic since they usually arise in the body.

3[55]. As far as the parturient is concerned, such are the causes of difficult labor; but as far as the child is concerned, they are the following: when it is extremely large, either in whole or in part, e.g. if it has a large head, or thorax, or a full belly, as it happens in those suffering from hydrocephalus. For not only normal children become large in their whole body or its parts, but abnormal ones as well. Moreover, difficult labor takes place on account of the number of children (when indeed there are two, both advancing at the same time, which become wedged in the neck of the uterus); or because the fetus is dead and does not co-operate in the delivery or, having died, has become swollen; or because of the abnormal position of the fetus. For the normal position for infants is head first, the hands stretched alongside the thighs, the fetus presenting in a straight line.[13] The following are abnormal positions: if, with the head bent to the side, the infant presses upon the right or left side of the uterus; or, if one or both hands protrude outside, while the legs within are parted from each other. Of the <remaining> positions, that with the feet first is the better, especially when the fetus presents in a straight line with the hands stretched alongside the thighs. Where one leg protrudes and the other remains inside, or where the infant is doubled up, or presses toward some part

[12] This again may be an allusion to a contracted pelvis, cf. above, p. 176.
[13] See Introduction, p. xlii.

of the uterus, correction is needed, as it is where the hands are extended upward.[14] Of the remaining two positions, the transverse [15] is the better one. Now there are three transverse positions: on either side, ⟨on the back,[16]⟩ on the abdomen. On the side is best, for it gives the hand of the midwife room to change the position either to head first or feet first. If the infant is doubled up, the worst position of all is present, particularly if presenting by the hips. For doubled-up infants can also assume three positions: since either the legs and the head are at the orifice of the uterus, or the abdomen, or the hips. It is better to have the abdomen toward the orifice of the uterus; for after we have opened the abdomen and removed its contents, the body collapses and it becomes easy to change the position.

Difficult labor also takes place if a monster has been conceived; furthermore, if the fetus has become denuded and the uterus is injured by the skeleton. The skeleton of the fetus is denuded if the flesh has rotted (which happens rarely), or often when the fetus is being inexpertly extracted, the flesh is torn off, and the bare bones injure the uterus.

4[56]. With regard to the birth passage, difficult labor takes place when the uterus has either a narrow orifice or a small one, or a small neck. Usually women who are of small stature have also a uterus in proportion to their other parts. Difficult labor also occurs because the neck of the uterus is bent, or because flesh has grown abnormally upon the neck or orifice of the uterus, or because there is inflammation, or

[14] We have kept the literal "hands" although "arms" might express the meaning more clearly.

[15] I.e. simple transverse.

[16] Ilberg, following Rose, conjectures *ischia,* i.e. hips. However, "back" seems a more satisfactory reading.

an abscess, or a scirrhus, or because the chorionic cloak is firm and the fetus unable to break it. Or, if the fluid that has gathered in the uterus is excreted before the proper time, the area remains without moisture and quite dry at the very time of birth, when there is need for this fluid to make a slippery and easy passage for the fetus.

A small orifice or small neck occurs for many reasons. For it obtains whenever women married before maturity conceive and give birth while the uterus has not yet fully grown nor the fundus of <the> uterus expanded. Difficult labor also takes place by reason of the peculiar nature of the constitution or makeup; for some women naturally have a small uterus, just as may be the case with any other part of the body. Furthermore, some women have difficult labor <because> they have conceived after prolonged widowhood, some because they are advanced in years and are weak, others because they deliver for the first time, are afraid, and ignorant of <the> proper position for their bodies. All these things are causes of difficult labor. Besides, difficulties arise from the pressure of faeces or urine, also if the parturient has a stone in the bladder, so that the neck of the uterus is compressed.

5[57].[17] Difficulties may also originate in the body from internal or external causes. This is the case when the parturient is very fleshy and very fat; or [because] the surrounding membrane [18] is difficult to break or does not contain sufficient fluid to effect slipperiness; or because the pubic bones have grown together, so that they are not capable of separating in parturition (for in women the <pubic bones> do not fuse into a solid joint as in men, but are bound to each other by a

[17] Ilberg, in the apparatus to this article, points out that the genuineness of the text appears uncertain.

[18] I.e. the chorion, according to Soranus.

strong ligament[19]); also because the region of the loin is too concave and exerts a lateral pressure upon the uterus.[20] Regarding causes outside the body, difficulties may arise for instance because the room has not been prepared beforehand; or because she is given to drink or late hours; or because the season is extremely cold and wintry (and the ducts narrowed thereby), or extremely hot and relaxing; or through the inexperience of the midwife or the physician. Moreover, difficult labor occurs, if in consequence of the pain the woman stretches violently or the chorion is torn away from <the> uterus, or compresses part of the uterus or falls forward entirely.[21] It also takes place because the blood is not carried through the uterus to the chorion but remains in the venous and arterial vessels which are implanted in the uterus, and dilates the vessels. Furthermore, as we have said,[22] difficult labor may be caused by any other pain. Such pain is sometimes associated with flatus, and the pangs of labor too are sometimes associated with flatus. <So says Demetrius the Herophilean.> No one has opposed or gainsaid him with regard to the causes just mentioned, but everyone has confirmed and supported him as one speaking truly; except that here again we might justly blame the Herophileans, because we contend that teleological faculties[23] have no place in a discussion of diseases;

19 According to the Hippocratic doctrine (as pointed out by Fasbender, *Entwickelungslehre,* p. 129 f.), the hip bones are separated in primiparae. Soranus (or rather Demetrius) seems the earliest author in whom we find the statement of the ligamentous symphysis in women.

20 The present passage has been tentatively interpreted by Fasbender, *Geschichte,* p. 43, as referring to scoliosis. See also above, p. 177.

21 This might be interpreted as referring to abruption of the placenta or placenta praevia.

22 It is not clear to what passage this refers.

23 Soranus refers to the "psychic" and "vital" faculties mentioned above in article 2. This doctrine of the "faculties" was elaborated by Galen, who distinguished "natural," "vital" and "psychic" faculties, and it remained

besides the Herophileans themselves do not agree as to their true nature.

How to diagnose the causes of difficult labor.

6[58]. Of the said causes of difficult labor some strike you by themselves, others do not. For excessive grief ⟨which⟩ renders the body loose and flabby, and the other psychic causes were discovered upon inquiry not to be conducive to easy labor. Torpor and lethargy [24] on the other hand are manifest causes; moreover, their signs can be learned from the book "On Acute Diseases." [25] We diagnose the size of the fetus as the cause of difficult labor from the largeness of the abdomen. If, however, the fetus advances and does not lighten the abdomen in proportion, one has to assume that there are plural infants. Moreover, we diagnose that the fetus is in transverse position, or has its hands thrown forward, in short, that the position is ⟨abnormal⟩, by insertion of the fingers. . . . For if it is alive, the parturient has labor pains and strains down, her ⟨abdomen is found⟩ warm ⟨and on insertion of⟩ the fingers the fetus itself is seen to be flushed.[26] But if it is dead, the parturient does not have pains in this manner and her abdomen is cold; ⟨and⟩ upon inserting the fingers the fetus appears to be neither warm nor gasping for breath; [27] moreover, if a part has prolapsed it is found black and necrotic. We diagnose an affected uterus by the touch,

---

dominant until the 16th century. It is worth noting, however, that apart from the philosophical objection, Soranus seems to accept Demetrius' doctrine in full.

24 On lethargy see above, pp. 158, 178 and corresponding footnotes.

25 Cf. Caelius Aurelianus, *Acute Dis.* II, ch. 3.

26 This is not clear; Soranus may refer to the appearance of a visible part.

27 This is the literal meaning of the term *asthmainon* which however *may* also mean "making an effort."

using the signs which have been mentioned in connection with its diseases.[28] If, however, something happens to the woman <during> parturition we recognize those who are in danger during childbirth from the pulse and respiration, and those who are lost from the disappearing pulse and the fact that they present signs of death.

II[XVIII]. *How in General to Treat Difficult Labor, and the Detailed Care of Difficult Labor.*

7[59]. In cases of difficult labor the physician should also question the midwife. <Now whether> it is caused by constriction and contraction of the region through which the fetus is to travel, or by coldness or heat of the atmosphere, or by hardness of the body, or because of a concavity of the loins,[29] or a naturally small uterus, or because of conceiving too early in life, or because of the burden of fat, or because of compressing tumors, or grief, or fear, or bending of the neck,[30] or inflammation or dryness, or whatever other cause, one should first promote ease and relaxation. And one should neither have immediate recourse to surgery nor allow the midwife long to dilate the uterus forcibly. Now if difficult labor takes place because the parturient has concave loins [31] one should place her upon her knees so that the uterus may fall toward the abdominal wall and come to lie in a straight line with its neck. Fat and very fleshy women should be placed similarly. If, however, the orifice of the uterus is closed, one should soften and relax it with greasy substances, i.e. one

[28] Cf. book III.
[29] Cf. above, pp. 177, 182.
[30] I.e. neck of the uterus.
[31] Cf. above, footnote 29.

should continually instill warm sweet olive oil, or combine it with a decoction of fenugreek or mallow or linseed and sometimes <the white> of eggs. For thus pressure is relieved while the difficult passages are moistened to slipperiness. Then one should also spread linseed or fenugreek in olive oil and hydromel over the pubes, the abdomen and loins, and should administer an oily sitz bath or fomentation with sea sponges, quickly wiping the moisture off with pieces of cloth. If patients are in pain, bladders <full> of warm olive oil should be applied or bags containing warm ground grain. Otherwise one may move them about on a litter in moderately warm air, the head of the patient somewhat raised, for slight movement stimulates expulsion. But some people have also employed vigorous shaking, for some have raised the legs of the bed at the head and, fastening the patient to the bedstead by means of a bandage around the chest, have ordered an assistant to lift the foot end of the bed with his hands and let it fall down to the floor.[32] <Others> have advised the ladder;[33] others have forced the patient to walk about; others to climb up and down steps; and still others have advised that somebody standing behind the parturient should put his hands under her armpits and lift and shake her vigorously. All such shaking must be rejected, for a shock to the uterus leads to ruptures and sympathetic reactions. One should use the previous instructions and should advise the parturient that she is in no danger and should take courage. Those who are not experienced in labor should be taught to hold the breath forcibly and press it toward the flanks. One should revive the woman

[32] A somewhat similar method in cases of difficult abortion is described in Hippocrates, "On Women's Diseases" I, 68 (ed. Littré, vol. 8, p. 142 ff.) under the name of "shaking."

[33] The method employed was possibly that of Euryphon in retention of the secundines; see book IV, 14; below, p. 197.

who has fainted with harmless ⟨things to smell⟩. A woman who is feeble because of prolonged illness should, during a short interval of relief,[34] be fed a little simple food (such as bread, melon, liquid barley gruel, apples and all similar things).[35] For there is a fear that, because of the excitement, a more abundant amount may be decomposed and altered.

Now under circumstances such as these, if the closed part has been opened by means of softening and greasy substances, one should also straighten the neck [36] if it is bent. One should push aside a tumor with ointment if it lies close by. If not, one should cut it out surgically whether it be a warty excrescence, or a calloused swelling, or a dividing membrane,[37] or a growth of flesh, or any other such obstacle. If the excreta have been kept back, one should get rid of the faeces by introducing an enema of water mixed with oil or hydromel, while the urine should be removed by means of the catheter if the bladder is full of urine. If a wedged-in stone is the cause, one must push the stone with the catheter out of the neck of the bladder and drive it back into the cavity. One should carefully cut through with the lancet a chorion that does not open, having first made a depression at some place with the finger. If, however, the fluid has already drained forth, one should instill some greasy fluid into the vagina by means of a small syringe.

8[60]. If the fetus is situated abnormally, one must make the position normal. If in a cephalic presentation the fetus lies out of position, one should introduce the anointed left

[34] I.e. relief from the pains of labor.

[35] In the Cod. Parisinus (see Ilberg's apparatus), these substances are mentioned as examples of what a fainting woman should be given to smell, and this is supported by Caelius Aurelianus, though not by Muscio.

[36] I.e. of the uterus.

[37] Cf. book I, 17.

hand, the nails being pared so that they may not scratch, and the fingers extended, joined together at their tips to give them a tapering shape so that they may be introduced without causing laceration. The hand should be inserted when the orifice of the uterus widens naturally, in order that this may not take place when it closes and contracts, creating a firm resistance. Having grasped the fetus, one should bring it into a straight line with the orifice of the uterus, assisting the change by making the parturient lie in the respective positions. For the patient must be placed on the opposite side: on the right side in those cases where the fetus is deviated to the left, but on the left side if the fetus has wandered to the right. She should lie back in a sloping position if the fetus has deviated forward as if against the abdominal wall, but should kneel forward with her face lowermost if the embryo has deviated inward as if against the loins. If, however, deviation is combined with impaction, one should first push up and lift the fetus, so that it is removed from the orifice of the uterus, and so straighten it. If, in addition, it has thrust out a hand, one should not seize it and pull (for impaction becomes greater when the head is bent further back or forward, or dislocation occurs; sometimes 〈even〉 dismemberment). 〈Instead〉 one should press with the finger tips against the shoulder and first push up the fetus, and when it is in the cavity [38] one should straighten it by bending the elbow and thus stretching the hand along the side and the thigh, so that delivery may be unhindered. If, moreover, the fetus has thrust out both hands, one should press with the finger tips against both shoulders and push it up; then one should push back the arms, bend the elbows towards the sides 〈and〉 stretch the hands along the thighs; and having got hold of

[38] I.e. of the uterus.

the infant's head, one should gently draw it out. In case the head happens to be small and the fetus has thrust out both hands, one should straighten the bent head, and having seized the hands, one should pull; for because of the smallness of the head, impaction sometimes does not take place.

If in a foot presentation the fetus is deviated in any direction, one must change its position and straighten it in much the same way as in cephalic presentation. In case it has thrust out one foot, one should again not grasp it and pull (for the fetus is further impacted by the other foot being bent). Instead, one should push with the finger tips against the region of the hip [39] and drive the fetus [40] back into the cavity of the uterus. Then, inserting the hand, one should straighten the other leg and stretch it out beside the first. ⟨If,⟩ however, the fetus has thrust out both feet while one or even both hands are bent backwards, one should again in like manner push up the fetus and put the hands aright. Where the feet are separated and press against different parts of the uterus, one has to bring them together ⟨and⟩ draw them in a straight line with the orifice of the uterus. If the fetus is presenting by the knees, one must push it up and when thus the legs have been straightened, one should extract it by the feet. If the buttocks present, one must also push the fetus up, then straighten the legs, and having put the hands along the thighs, one should extract it by the feet.

Moreover, if the fetus lies in a transverse position,[41] whether with its face downwards ⟨or⟩ on its back, one should gently turn it over on its side with the fingers so that there may be space to insert the hand. If the fetus is spontaneously

[39] I.e. of the infant. For the Greek text of this passage, see F. Ernst Kind, Zu Sorans Repositionstechnik des vorgefallenen Fusses, in *Sudhoffs Archiv für Geschichte der Medizin,* 1939, vol. 32, pp. 333–336.

[40] See Kind, *ibid.*

[41] Cf. p. 180.

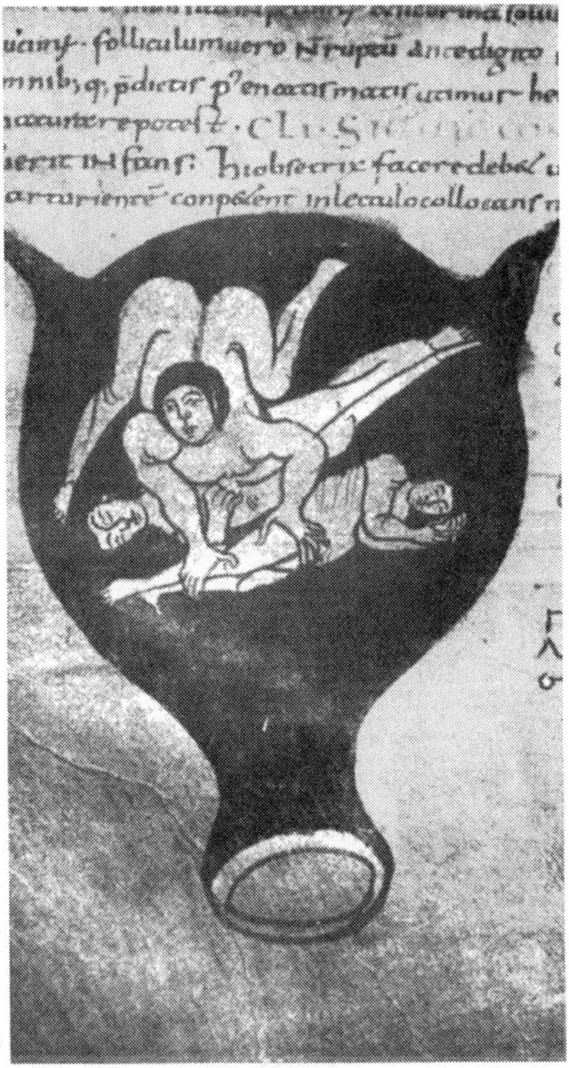

FIGURE 2 *Positions of the fetus. Illustration accompanying a Muscio text of about 900* A.D. *(Brussels MS. 3714; see Introduction, p. xliii).*

lying on its side, one must put in the hand by the side and gently turn it [42] . . . . For the position on the head is better since the broad parts pass through first and the hands are not bent further back. If, however, the fetus is doubled up, the doubled part lying upwards while the extremities lie evenly alongside of one another, one must straighten it having first pushed the legs up. If, however, it is not doubled up evenly, one must first turn it over and make the doubled part lie towards the fundus; then after turning, as we have said, one should straighten it. If more than one fetus present, one must push them up again, turn them in the direction of the cavity and deliver them one at a time. One should do everything gently and without bruising, and should continually anoint the parts with oil, so that the parturient remains free from sympathetic trouble and the infant healthy; for we see many alive who have thus been born with difficulty.

III[XIX]. *On Extraction by Hooks and Embryotomy.*

9[61]. If the fetus does not respond to manual traction, because of its size, or death, or impaction in any manner

[42] The rest of the sentence is interrupted by a lacuna and its meaning, therefore, is obscure and has been left untranslated. From the passage in Caelius Aurelianus, *Gynaecia* (p. 102, 1093), it can be inferred that Soranus dealt with two possibilities. If the position is oblique, then the parts further away from the orifice should be brought in line with those closer to the orifice. If it is transverse then delivery by the head, if possible, should be aimed at. The whole paragraph in the *Gynaecia* (1090–98) reads: "at si oblicus venerit, vel supinus vel pronus, erit sensim supra latus vertendus, quo immittende manui detur locus. set si supra latus veniens descenderit, immissa manu sensim erit vertendus. set si iniquum erit partium libramentum, ut altera pars ori matricis plus ab altera vicinetur, erit magis interiori favendum ut sue exterior correctioni consentiat. si vero obliquitas fuerit equalis, ut in partita corporis longitudine ori matricis medium videatur obiectum, erit melius, si fieri potest, caput prius in exitum provocare." Cf. also Muscio, p. 88 f.

whatsoever, one must proceed to the more forceful methods, those of extraction by hooks and embryotomy. For even if one loses the infant, it is still necessary to take care of the mother. Therefore, one should warn of the underlying danger of supervening fevers, sympathetic nervous troubles, sometimes even of excessive inflammation, and that there is little hope particularly if gangrene appears; in the latter case, there is weakening, profuse perspiration, chills, imperceptible pulse, sharp fever, delirium and convulsions.

Nevertheless, one should not withhold assistance. ⟨Now one should⟩ put the whole patient in a sloping position ⟨upon a bed⟩ which is relatively hard, so that the loins are not allowed to sink in. With the thighs parted and drawn towards the abdomen, she should prop herself with her feet against the bedstead. Then one should have her held fast on either side by servants; but if such are not present, one should fasten down her thorax to the bed by means of a bandage, so that the body of the patient cannot follow the extraction of the fetus and thus lessen the force of the pull. The physician himself should sit down opposite and a little lower so that his hands are on the same level as the feet of the patient. The labia being parted to either side by servants, he should again insert the left hand (because it is softer than the right one and can more effectively be introduced with delicacy) [43] with the fingers anointed and joined together at the tips to give them a tapering shape. This he should do if the orifice of the uterus is open, but otherwise after it has been relaxed by means of pressure and continuous anointing with oil. Then one should try if possible to make straight what is deviated and should seek a place for the insertion of the hook so that it may not easily fall out.

[43] See pp. 194, 195.

10[62]. In cephalic presentation, places suitable for inserting it [44] are the eyes, the back of the head, the roof of the mouth, the collarbones and the area below the ribs. The armpits, however, are in no wise suitable (for if during extraction the arms are further abducted, the circumference of the fetus is increased so as to lead to impaction); nor are the auditory canals suitable (since they hardly admit the hook, because of their crookedness, and are too narrow). In foot presentation, the bones above the pudenda, the spaces between the ribs and the clavicular [45] region are suitable. But in case none of the said places is found, an incision with a knife is to be made for the insertion.

One should hold the hook, previously warmed in olive oil, with the right hand. Covering its curvature with the fingers, one should gently introduce it with the help of the left hand and insert it into any of the said places until it has penetrated deeply. One should also insert a second hook, opposite the first, so that traction may be evenly balanced and not one-sided, causing a part to deviate and consequently impaction of the fetus. Next one should give an experienced person the hooks to hold with the admonition that he pull the fetus gently with them, without tearing it to pieces by pulling, nor on the other hand, letting it go (for if relaxed, the part that has emerged slips back). Rather, when it is necessary to pause in the traction, he should keep the hooks at the previous tension. Nor should he pull only in a straight line, but should also deviate to the sides in the manner done in extracting teeth. For if the position of the fetus is thus changed by the levering motion, it widens the region and will be easily

[44] I.e. the hook.

[45] The word for "clavicular region," *katakleis,* is not certain in its meaning; see below, p. 193, where it has been translated by "clavicle." Other suggestions include "acromion" and "first rib."

extracted. While the physician is in this manner skilfully assisted, he should introduce between the orifice of the uterus and the impacted body his forefinger, moving it around in a circle as if stripping a skin off, and straightening what is displaced to one side. Moreover, he should thoroughly anoint the region with warm olive oil or any of the slippery decoctions that have been mentioned.[46] If, nevertheless, the fetus does not at once respond to the pull of the hooks and emerge, but moves little by little along with each pull, the physician will have to insert <the> first hook again into parts which lie higher up, then the second hook, and so on, until the whole body of the fetus has passed through. In foot presentation, he should proceed in like manner.

11[63]. If, however, a hand has prolapsed and cannot be turned back because of the severe impaction, or if the fetus is already dead (as we conjecture from the fact that the part is neither flushed nor warm nor pulsating but livid, cold and without pulsation), one should throw a piece of cloth over it to prevent slipping and draw it forward slightly. Then depressing it in order that the parts lying above may become more visible, one should amputate at the shoulder joint. The same should be done if a leg has prolapsed. Then one should turn [47] the rest of the body with the fingers and deliver by inserting the hooks. If both hands have fallen forward and cannot be turned back nor disengaged by pulling, one must remove them both by cutting them off at the shoulders, as has been done with one hand. If, however, the impaction is caused by too big a head, and if the fetus suffers from hydrocephalus,

[46] Cf. p. 184 f.

[47] The meaning is not quite clear. The word may connote a turning around of the infant or merely pushing it back.

one should split it with an embryotome or a knife for removing polypi, covered during its introduction between the forefinger and the little finger, so that the fluid may be emptied and the circumference of the head collapse. If, however, the fetus naturally has a large head, one should crush the head with the hand, <for> it yields easily when the body is still soft. Otherwise, it is well to lay open the skull with the knife either at the bregma or, if this is not possible, at any other place. For after the brain has been cleared out, the head collapses. The edges of the incision must be turned aside and the little bones fragmented by means of a forceps for drawing teeth, or a forceps for extracting splinters of bone. If, however, because of the large size of the whole body, the fetus does not respond even if so pulled, the shoulders arrested by the lateral parts of the uterus, one must plunge the knife into the jugular region until it has penetrated deeply into the fetus. For when the blood is drained off, the body becomes thin. Afterwards one should lay open the whole head and also cut through the intercostal spaces and <the> lungs. For the latter are often full of fluid and have distended the thorax. One should also free <the> parts of the chest which are bound to one another by tearing away with the fingers the clavicles from the sternum [48] <or>, if they <do not> yield, one should break them off. For the chest collapses when its parts are no longer held apart by the so-called collarbones. But if even so the fetus does not respond one should perforate the abdomen; and should do likewise if the fetus is dropsical. For when the fluid is emptied, the circumference

[48] The translations of "clavicles" (*katakleis,* pl.) and "sternum" (*antisternon,* pl.) are questionable, since the meaning of the Greek words is fluctuating. See also p. 191.

of the body collapses and is reduced. In case the intestines too have contributed to the swelling of the abdomen, one must first draw them out together with the other adjacent viscera and thus deliver the whole body.

12[64]. The same should also be done in foot presentations. If, in addition, the hands are bent upwards, one should amputate; and if the head is too big, again one should crush it. However, in such a position this is more difficult, because the head is hidden high up. It will be necessary to seize the feet with the right hand and pull, and with the left hand straighten the head from inside. For when the latter is bent back upon the isthmus of the uterus, it is often torn off. It is, however, hard to understand why the left hand should be appropriate for pulling and to explain it on the grounds that serpents too are lifted with it—for both statements are wrong.[49] Contrariwise it is especially suitable to introduce, as we have shown above.[50]

If the fetus is in transverse position or is folded up, and cannot be straightened, one should cut into the parts which are presenting—in some cases the abdomen, in others the armpits, the intercostal spaces, or the region of the kidneys in the direction of the flanks. If the fetus is dead and of excessive size, it is dangerous to morcellate it entirely within the uterus. It is better to cut each of the parts as it presents. In these cases amputations at the joints are indicated, for at their ends even the bones are easily freed from their connections. But it is necessary to put together the removed parts and to pay heed lest ⟨any⟩ have been left behind. Often, however, because of the traction exerted upon the feet by

[49] As Pliny, xxviii, 33, shows, there really existed such a belief with regard to snakes ("serpentis aegre praeterquam laeva manu extrahi").

[50] Cf. above, p. 190.

inexperienced persons, the head is torn off and is hard to grasp because of its rounded shape and because it slips away into the uterine cavity. In such cases, just as in stones of the bladder, Sostratus introduces the finger of the left hand into the anus [51] while pressing with the right hand upon the abdomen, and tries to bring down the head. He does not see that in the rectum <the> finger cannot reach the head. For whereas the bladder is readily accessible, the uterus extends far beyond, as we have shown above.[52] Therefore, having introduced the hand and touched the head, one should make the latter descend by rotation as far as the neck of the uterus, and should then deliver it by inserting a hook. But if the orifice is closed, one must proceed as we shall indicate in connection with the afterbirth.[53]

13[65]. After extraction by hooks and embryotomy, since the region is already inflamed because of the ensuing irritation, one should induce relaxation and soothe by means of embrocations. If hemorrhage has occurred, one should use things appropriate to it.

But to prescribe in addition drugs promoting quick birth, as did the followers of Hippocrates among others, is without foundation.[54] For neither dried leaves of sweet bay in warm water, nor dittany or southernwood and cedar resin, and anise with sweet old olive oil, nor the fruit of the wild cucumber

51 According to Celsus VII, 26, 2 E, the surgeon in lithotomy introduces first the index finger, then the middle finger of the left hand into the anus. Paul of Aegina, VI, 60, makes the surgeon introduce the left index finger if the patient is a child, and the left middle finger as well, if an adult.

52 Cf. book I, 7.

53 Literally: *chorion;* cf. below, p. 199.

54 Cf. Hippocrates, "On Women's Diseases" I, 77 (ed. Littré, vol. 8, pp. 170–172) where all the drugs mentioned in the following sentence are recommended as promoting quick birth, although the mode of preparation differs somewhat.

added to a date salve [55] and fastened upon the loins effect quick birth. Whereas the above-mentioned treatment removes the morbid condition and thus also removes the resulting ill effect.

IV[XX]. *On Retention of the Secundines.*

14[I 71]. After delivery of the fetus the chorion which <indeed> is also called "secundine" [56] is often left behind and makes trouble by affecting the uterus and causing the latter to contract about it. And because of this, it produces pain in the head and lower abdomen, and convulsions or suffocation. Sometimes the connection with the umbilicus of the fetus is still preserved, sometimes it is torn off (when the fetus drops unexpectedly or when the midwife has torn it off inexpertly), sometimes the chorion is hidden from sight, while at other times it is partially extruded. And the connection or attachment with the uterus is either still preserved or loosened, while the orifice of the uterus is sometimes closed, sometimes still open, and inflammation is either absent or present.

Now Hippocrates [57] uses sternutatives and draws together the nostrils so that the afterbirth [58] may be driven out by the descending pressure of the breath.[59] Euryphon, the Cni-

[55] A cerate which has juice from the date tree, probably the efflorescences, as an ingredient. See Galen, ed. Kühn, vol. 13, 375 ff. where he describes his mode of preparing the "date" plaster.

[56] Cf. book I, 57, above p. 58, whence it is evident that by "chorion" or "secundines" Soranus here includes the whole placenta.

[57] Cf. Hippocrates, "Aphorisms" V, 49: "To expel the after-birth: apply something to cause sneezing and compress the nostrils and the mouth" (ed. Jones, vol. 4, p. 171). See also "Epidemics" II, 5, 25 (ed. Littré, vol. 5, p. 132).

[58] Literally: *chorion.*

[59] Cf. the recent practice of "quilling."

dian,[60] however, employs diuretic potions made from dittany and salvia, and blood-drawing suppositories made of soapwort, Illyrian iris, cantharides and honey. Also he employs shaking by means of a ladder to which the patient has been bound. Euenor and Sostratus and Apollonius, the Prusian, say that it is necessary to grasp the projecting part and thus draw the chorion out. Dion gives draughts prepared with salvia, myrrh, and celery seed. Some people fumigate with such substances as bitumen, human hair, hartshorn, galbanum, black cummin or wormwood. Straton, the Erasistratean, puts aromatic herbs, such as spikenard and cassia, furthermore horehound, wormwood, dittany, oil of lilies and roses, and honey into a silver or copper pot which has been lined with tin. Then he takes hold of the lid, puts a pipe around, the other end of which he fits into the vagina, and foments the region by warming the vessel over a small fire.[61] Mantias, however, puts the infant upon the thighs of the parturient so that the afterbirth [62] may thus be drawn forward by the natural movements of the infant itself. If the connection of the afterbirth [62] with the infant is not preserved, he suspends a large piece of lead from the protruding part, so that the afterbirth [62] may be drawn forward by the weight.[63]

15[I 72]. All the aforesaid things are bad. For the in-

60 Prescriptions reminiscent of those ascribed to Euryphon are listed in Hippocrates, "On Women's Diseases" I, 78 (ed. Littré, vol. 8, p. 176 ff.) and "On the Nature of Women" 32 (ed. Littré, vol. 7, p. 346 ff.).

61 A similar apparatus for vaginal fumigations in prolapse of the uterus is described in detail by Antyllus (Oribasius, *Collect. med.* x, 19; vol. 2, p. 425 f.).

62 Literally: *chorion.*

63 Hippocrates, "On Superfetation," ch. 8 (ed. Littré, vol. 8, p. 480 f.) describes a method whereby the child (or a weight) is placed below the sitting mother and its weight is allowed gradually to increase the pull.

creased agitation produced by sternutatives causes danger of immediate hemorrhage or of later nervous sympathetic reactions. The draughts harm the stomach and upset it, while the blood-drawing vaginal suppositories are irritating and ulcerating and thereby cause convulsions, spasms and sympathetic reactions. Shaking causes violent agitation. Any pulling on the afterbirth,[64] because of the agitation, leads to inflammation, and is, moreover, impossible in cases where the orifice is closed and no part of the afterbirth [64] protrudes. Fumigations increase inflammation by their pungency and cause congestion in the head. For the same reason, fomentation with aromatic herbs is futile; moreover, if the pipe whose other end is placed in the vagina becomes hot by transmission of the heat, it burns the parts. It is also hurtful to drag away forcibly the protruding part by suspending lead, especially if inflammation is already present. If the string is but weakly tied to the afterbirth[64] it will slip off altogether, and if it is tied strongly, it will cause sympathetic reactions and fainting. Besides, ⟨a part⟩ of the afterbirth [64] does not always protrude. Likewise, extraction by the movements of the child is dangerous, for the traction must be carried out expertly.

16[I 73]. Therefore, if the connection of the afterbirth with the umbilicus is still preserved, the infant should be placed with a cloth under it upon the hands of one woman servant. Then, guided somehow by the cord [65] that grows to the umbilicus, one must insert the hand ⟨and⟩, while the parturient strains, one should gently remove the afterbirth [66] by lateral movements without rending and tearing it. If, however, the procedure requires more time, one should re-

[64] Literally: *chorion.*
[65] Literally: "The intestine that is like the *ourachos*"; cf. book I, 57.
[66] Literally: *chorion.*

lease the infant from its attachment, but otherwise do the same. If it is not attached at all,[67] one must take the infant away and then it will be best to grasp the protruding part and deliver gently, relaxing when the orifice contracts, pulling when it widens. If no part protrudes and the orifice remains distended, one should insert the anointed hand and, if the afterbirth[68] is free from its attachment to the uterus and folded on itself, one should grasp it and pull. If, however, it is attached, one should spread out the fingers and should try to free it gently from inside by working around from side to side. For those men, who through lack of experience pull in a straight line, have often by their pulling even caused inversion of the uterus. But if the secundines do not yield to relatively gentle traction, or in case the orifice is closed and inflamed,[69] one should leave them alone and treat as an inflammation with injections and poulticing of the organs and with warm food; for when the inflammation ceases, the foreign body is set free and falls out in a state of mortification. (In this manner sometimes a dislocated limb has been kept out by the fluid, <but>, with the inflammation gone, has yielded to reduction).[70] Unless the roots of scrofulous glands are attached, some people wait for future mortification.[71] But an afterbirth[72] that is attached to the viscus[73] by means of blood vessels must be forcibly detached and not

[67] It is not quite clear whether Soranus thinks of the attachment of the umbilical cord to the placenta, or of the placenta to the uterus.

[68] Literally: *chorion.*

[69] This points to a late summoning of the physician consultant who finds the cervix already contracted.

[70] The simile seems to point to the difficulty of setting a dislocated limb while inflammation and periarticular fluids abound.

[71] The meaning is unclear possibly due to corruption of the text.

[72] Literally: *chorion.*

[73] I.e. the uterus.

left till it relaxes and can be removed gently because of the putrefaction.

v[xxi]. ⟨*On Abscesses in the Female Genitals.*⟩ [74]

vi[xxii]. ⟨*On Ulcers of the Uterus.*⟩

vii[xxiii]. ⟨*On Cancers in the Uterus.*⟩

viii[xxiv]. ⟨*On Fistulas in the Uterus.*⟩

ix[xxv]. ⟨*On Enlarged Clitoris.*⟩

x[xxvi]. ⟨*On Cercosis.*⟩

xi[xxvii]. ⟨*On Warty Excrescences in the Female Genitals.*⟩

xii[xxviii]. ⟨*On Fissures.*⟩

xiii[xxix]. ⟨*On Knobby Swellings.*⟩

xiv[xxx]. ⟨*On Hemorrhoids in the Uterus.*⟩

xv[xxxi]. *On Prolapse of the Uterus.*

35[84]. The dangerous condition of partial eversion of the uterus is called prolapse of the uterus; for the uterus, if loosened from the attachments, does not, as some people as-

[74] For the approximate content of the missing ten chapters the English reader is referred to the respective chapters in Adams' translation of Paul of Aegina and Ricci's *Aetios of Amida* (see Introduction, p. xlix). Paul of Aegina, vi, 70 (Adams' translation, ii, p. 381), defines "cercosis" as "a fleshy excrescence arising from the mouth of the womb, and filling the female pudendum, sometimes even projecting externally like a tail."

sume, prolapse as a whole,[75] (indeed <when such a complete> prolapse <occurs>, it cannot be restored). The prolapsing part is similar to the egg of an ostrich and is bigger or smaller in proportion to the force with which the eversion is produced. The uterus prolapses rarely, yet the causes may be several. Thus a woman who falls from a height and lands on the hips suffers it, if certain membranes [76] connecting the uterus with its neighboring parts are ruptured <and torn off>. It also occurs because of a vigorous extraction of the chorion, and happens particularly in the so-called premature births. Unskilful extraction of the fetus by hooks has also caused the disorder. It is brought about, moreover, through holding <the> breath, or leaping, and from lifting a weight, or from a blow; sometimes also because of the application of much viscous fluid <if, from much moisture, the ligaments of the upper part of the fundus of the uterus become relaxed and weakened>. But it has also occurred through mental stress; for when the loss of children or the approach of enemies was announced, or when women were exposed to severe storms at sea, they suffered a prolapse, their whole physique being relaxed, so that the uterus slipped out. Sometimes the disorder has come about without any such cause, the body being weakened and the membranes and muscles supporting the uterus likewise being relaxed by weakness, as happens in women past their prime. Now in the beginning there is considerable bleeding; then, in addition, pain in the flanks, loins, the abdomen and the pudenda, and there is danger of supervening convulsion when <the parts> are cooled down. When the condition has become chronic and the prolapsed body has grown calloused, danger and pain are removed.

[75] Cf. book I, 13, above, p. 12.
[76] I.e. ligaments.

36[85]. Some say that the whole uterus prolapses [77] if the membranes and muscles which support it are ruptured by a blow or anything similar <or> become relaxed and suffer something like paralysis. But the followers of Hippocrates [78] and Herophilus say that the orifice only prolapses (it is recognized by the softness, the prolapsing body being similar to the head of an octopus, as Herophilus said,[79] and having a duct which will admit a probe). Others say that the uterus does not prolapse at all, for in their opinion no part of the uterus slips down; rather, the inflamed orifice gives the impression of a prolapse. Still others maintain that the prolapse of the uterus takes place in the manner of an eversion, so that sometimes its outer covering prolapses, sometimes the inner. For they say that the uterus has two coverings and that its outer covering is attached to the parts above, while the inner covering is joined to it, and that prolapse occurs because of the relaxation of the membranes. Again others maintain that the uterus may prolapse as a whole because of a rupture or weakness, or in part, and may furthermore fold up into its own cavity. Now when it prolapses because of a rupture caused by a fall or some violence or a blow, they say it will appear bloody from first to last. But when it prolapses because of looseness or even paralysis, it will appear neither bloody nor thickened; in most cases the paralysis is from an unknown cause, sometimes, however, from conditions like the forementioned. If, on the other hand, the uterus has prolapsed

[77] A total prolapse of the uterus is described in Hippocrates, "On Women's Diseases" II, 144 (ed. Littré, vol. 8, p. 316): "If the uterus falls entirely out of the vagina, it is suspended like a scrotum. Pain seizes the lower abdomen, the waist and the groins." (Similarly, vol. 7, p. 316 f. and vol. 8, p. 460).

[78] Ilberg refers to Hippocrates, ed. Littré, vol. 8, p. 318 ff. But there is no statement there that the orifice only prolapses.

[79] Cf. book I, 10 (end).

in part, protruding parts may be seen on each side as in the case of the rectum. In case of an inversion of <the> whole circumference, a round mass is found prolapsing, resembling an egg; sometimes it remains in the vagina, sometimes it projects further, even in front of the labia. It is reddish in the beginning, but whitish later on.

Even granting that the uterus may slip down as a whole <or> in part, we censure first of all Euryphon who makes <the> patient hang by her feet from a ladder for a whole day and night and then, making her lie down on her back, feeds her cold barley juice.[80] For the suspension is unbearable, the food causes flatulence and the computation of the days by which he calculates the proper time,[81] is not in accordance with the art. Euenor inserts ox meat into the vagina not knowing that the ichors produced by the putrefaction will, by their pungency, cause ulcerations. Diocles in the second book "On Gynecology," adjusts the uterus by forcing air in by means of a blacksmith's bellows, and afterwards dips peeled pomegranates into vinegar and inserts them. Thus he causes colic with the air and bruising with the pomegranate, for the latter is rough and astringent. Some people apply a hairy bag to the uterus, so that the organ may suffer pain from the sharp hair and contract. They are not aware that paralyzed parts do not suffer any pain while parts that feel pain contract for a little while and prolapse again. But the majority administer pleasant aromas to smell, while they apply fumigations to the uterus of an opposite character;

[80] A similar treatment is described in Hippocrates, "On Women's Diseases" III, 248 (ed. Littré, vol. 8, p. 462; cf. also *ibid.* p. 318 and vol. 7, p. 318), where the suspension on the ladder is probably limited to the short period of manual reposition of the uterus (see Ilberg, p. 149, notes).

[81] This may refer, as Ilberg thinks, to the treatment as detailed in Hippocrates, ed. Littré, vol. 8, p. 318.

and they believe that now the uterus like an animal flees the bad odors and turns towards the good ones.[82] We also censure Straton who fills the vagina with moistened ashes and uses a suppository of castoreum; for the ashes are pungent and the castoreum causes congestion.

37[86]. If the prolapse is fresh and the uterus looks bloody and not inflamed, it is best to rinse the organ first with cold water or diluted vinegar and to undertake the adjustment of it with the fingers; for in the beginning, the uterus easily yields to the reduction. If, however, it does not yield, one should adjust it by the application of a round sea sponge, while <the thighs> are lifted by some persons capable of assisting dexterously. After the adjustment one should fill the vagina with an inserted piece of sea sponge soaked in diluted vinegar or a piece of wool, and having fastened it with a bandage one should bring the thighs together and tie [83] them in an extended position. One should lift the region of the loin by placing a cushion underneath, or raise the lower end of the bed. Moreover, the patient should be made to fast until the third day and then given a little simple food, and every other day thereafter. When the adjustment has become fixed, one should carefully restore the strength [84] . . . if the age is taken into consideration. [87]. For in older women the uterus is adjustable, but readily prolapses again.

38. If impacted faeces lie in the rectum, they should be removed by a simple enema. Likewise, if there is any residuum in the bladder, it should be removed by a catheter. For it usually happens that these substances are held back because

[82] Cf. book III, 29.

[83] May also mean "cross them."

[84] I.e. prescribe the "restorative" treatment. The following lacuna disconnects the rest of the paragraph.

the uterus is situated between the rectum and the bladder, <and> when prolapsed forms an obstacle to natural evacuation, bruising and compressing those organs, <while its reduction is hindered by them>. Afterwards the patient should be placed upon her back with the hips elevated and the popliteal region bent while the legs are separated. Then for a long time one should bathe the prolapsed part of the uterus with much lukewarm olive oil, and make a woolen tampon corresponding in shape and diameter to the vagina and wrap it in very thin clean linen. Afterwards one should dip it briefly in diluted vinegar or the juice of acacia or of hypocist mixed with wine, apply it to the uterus and move the whole prolapsed part, forcing it up gently until the uterus has reverted to its proper place and the whole mass of wool is in the vagina. Then one should make an external application of wool soaked in astringent wine and afterwards cover the entire lower abdomen with a sea sponge or wool squeezed in diluted vinegar. Next one should cover the abdomen, pubes and loin as well, bandage them and extend the legs of the woman so that one lies on top of the other. Afterwards cupping vessels with a considerable flame are to be applied near the umbilicus on each flank, and sweet-smelling aromas held to the nostrils continuously.[85] On the third day, the woman with the wool remaining in the vagina ought to take a sitz bath in dark tart wine which has been slightly warmed or in a decoction of bramble or myrtle or mastich or pomegranate peel. After the sitz bath, she should lie down on her back in a tilted position, so that the region of the hips is higher up; the inserted wool should be taken out and another piece soaked in the same medicine put in. The abdomen should be poulticed with dates, barley

85 This application of aromatics has no rational explanation.

groats, pomegranate peel, <and lentils with oxymel>. And every third day the same should be repeated until the cure is complete.

39[88]. If, however, the uterus has remained outside for a long time and already looks whitish and seems cooled, or sometimes manifestly inflamed and painful, or if it seems to have prolapsed from paralysis, <one should bathe> it with warm water or oil mixed with water, or the juice of boiled fenugreek, or of linseed or mallow and thus reduce it. But if the amount <of inflammation> requires it one should bleed and use other relaxing remedies because of the paralysis. If, however, the condition is chronic so that the uterus prolapses constantly, one should wash it thoroughly with warm diluted vinegar and give a sitz bath of diluted vinegar for a long enough time. Then one should employ all the forementioned things,[86] that is: dry cupping, plasters with dates, quinces and everything that has an astringent effect or willow plasters and things which have the same action. Afterwards one ought to tone up the whole body by using the restorative cycle and subsequently the metasyncritic cycle; [87] one should irritate the pubic region, the loins and the abdomen with intense heat, pungent unctions, mustard plasters, vaginal suppositories containing natron, raisins <and> salt, and everything that is prepared from metasyncritic substances. But the majority sprinkle the continually prolapsing uterus with salt or natron, and thus push it back, a practice also adopted by Thessalus though <not> in accord with his own doctrines. For metasyncritic remedies must be employed during a remission rather than during the exacerbation when the uterus is prolapsed.

40[89]. If part of the uterus has turned black because

[86] Cf. the preceding article.
[87] Cf. Introduction, p. xxxv.

of having remained outside for a long time, and despite the statement [88] that in some women prolapse of the uterus has accompanied them to the grave, one must employ the remedies used for ulceration. Otherwise one should cut off the black part, considering the fact that we also cut away a lobe [89] of the liver or of the lung when it has turned black in cases of their protrusion.[90] If the whole uterus has become black, one must cut it off in its entirety, not only because of those who have related that it can be excised without danger and whom we mentioned before,[91] but because the part which is being amputated is no longer important but has become a foreign and unrelated body. In case the uterus has become ulcerated from constant prolapse and has grown to the labia as some people relate, one must sever the adhesion, like an adhesion of the intestine to the peritoneum. However, for safety's sake it is better to sacrifice a little of the labia in favor of the uterus if the division cannot be accomplished evenly.

XVI[XXXII]. ⟨*On Phimosis of the Uterus.*⟩

XVII[XXXIII]. ⟨*On Atresia.*⟩

XVIII[XXXIV]. ⟨*On the Use of the Speculum.*⟩

[88] Literally: "even if some people relate."
[89] "Lobe" may simply mean "a part."
[90] This analogy probably refers to post-traumatic herniation of the organs.
[91] Cf. book I, 15.

ANCIENT NAMES

MATERIA MEDICA

INDEX OF PERSONAL NAMES AND SUBJECTS

ANCIENT NAMES *

ALEXANDER PHILALETHES: Flourished about the time of the emperor Augustus and was head of a school of Herophilean physicians located between Laodiceia and Carura in Asia Minor.

ANDREAS: Possibly identical with the famous pharmacologist Andreas who lived in the later 3rd century B.C. The addressee of his book "To Sobios" is unknown.

ANTIGENES: Probably a pupil of Cleophantus (q.v.); 3rd century B.C.

APOLLONIUS BIBLAS: According to M. Wellmann (in *Pauly-Wissowa*), Apollonius called Biblas was a physician from Antioch who lived in the 2nd century B.C. and belonged to the empirical sect. Cf. Deichgräber, *Empirikerschule*, pp. 172 and 257.

APOLLONIUS MYS: Follower of Herophilus, lived about the time of the emperor Augustus. The book "On the Sect" dealt with the sect of Herophilus (Caelius Aurelianus, *Acute Dis.* II, 88, 13: "item Apollonius qui appellatus est Mys, volumine vicesimo octavo quod De secta Herophili conscripsit").

APOLLONIUS THE PRUSIAN: Otherwise unknown.

ARISTANAX: Otherwise unknown.

ARISTOTLE: Philosopher and scientist (384–322 B.C.).

ASCLEPIADES: Contemporary of Cicero (1st century B.C.); see Introduction, p. xxvi.

ATHENION: Follower of Erasistratus, lived after 250 B.C.

CEPHISOPHON: Author of a cataplasm named after him.

CLEOPHANTUS: Brother of Erasistratus (q.v.) flourished in Alexandria, 3rd century B.C. Wrote, among others, a comprehensive work "On Gynecology" quoted by Soranus.

DAMASTES: This Damastes is otherwise unknown, although Diels, *Die*

* This index lists the names of persons mentioned by Soranus in his *Gynecology*.

Handschriften der antiken Aerzte, 2. Teil, Berlin, 1906, p. 26, cites a Greek manuscript of the 11th century "On the Treatment of Pregnant Women and of Infants" by one Damnastes.

DEMETRIUS: Soranus mentions (a) Demetrius of Apamea, identical with the author of the book on "Semeiotics" (Caelius Aurelianus, *Chronic Dis.* v, 89: "Demetrius Apameus libro Signorum") and (b) Demetrius the Herophilean who, according to Caelius Aurelianus (*Acute Dis.* I, 4; II, 141; *Chronic Dis.* III, 99), wrote a work on pathology in many books. This Demetrius must have lived some time after 250 B.C. It is not certain whether the two are identical.

DEMOCRITUS: Philosopher, one of the founders of the ancient atomistic system, born in Abdera, lived in the 5th century B.C. For an English translation of the fragments of his writings, see Freeman, *Ancilla,* pp. 91–120.

DIOCLES THE CARYSTEAN: Famous physician who lived in the 4th century B.C.; cf. Werner Jaeger, *Diokles von Karystos,* Berlin, De Gruyter, 1938. The fragments of his works, including those of his "Gynecology," have been collected in Wellmann, *Fragmente.*

DION: Oribasius (ed. Bussemaker et Daremberg, vol. 5, p. 137) mentions an eye-salve by one Dion. Otherwise unknown.

DIONYSIUS: Probably the methodist physician who, according to Pseudo-Galen (ed. Kühn, vol. 14, p. 684), lived after Themison and Thessalus, i.e. in the later part of the 1st century A.D. His adherence to the methodist sect is also indicated by his relation to Mnaseas.

EMPEDOCLES: Empedocles of Agrigentum, 5th century B.C., pre-Socratic philosopher who originated the theory of fire, water, air, and earth as the roots of all things. For an English translation of the fragments of his writings see Freeman, *Ancilla,* pp. 51–69; also, *The Fragments of Empedocles,* translated into English verse by William Ellery Leonard, Chicago, 1908.

ERASISTRATUS: Anatomist and physician, flourished in Alexandria in the first half of the 3rd century B.C. According to Erasistratus, all tissues consisted of a net of arteries, veins, and nerves with a *parenchyma* in between. Followers of Erasistratus still existed in the 2nd century A.D.

EUDEMUS: Probably the Alexandrian anatomist who was a younger contemporary of Erasistratus and Herophilus (3rd century B.C.).

EUENOR: Physician, flourished in the second half of the 4th century B.C.

EURYPHON THE CNIDIAN: Older contemporary of Hippocrates. His views often resemble those found in the gynecological works of the Hippocratic collection.

HERON: Alexandrian surgeon mentioned by Celsus, VII, preface and ch. 14.

HEROPHILUS: Born in Chalcedon, Bithynia, flourished in Alexandria in the first half of the 3rd century B.C., anatomist and physician; little is known of his book "Against the Common Dogmas." His "Midwifery" formed an important gynecological source for later physicians, including Soranus. Followers of his sect still existed at Soranus' time. Cf. J. F. Dobson, Herophilus of Alexandria, *Proceed. of the Royal Soc. of Med.* 1925, vol. XVIII (Section Hist. of Med.), pp. 19–32.

HIPPOCRATES: Of Cos, contemporary of Socrates. The collection of medical works preserved under his name comprises books by different authors, the majority of whom lived around 400 B.C. Of the books of this collection Soranus mentions by title "Aphorisms" and "On the Nature of the Child."

LUCIUS: A physician of this name, author of a work on "Chronic Diseases" is mentioned by Caelius Aurelianus (*Chronic Dis.* II, 59 and 111; IV, 78). He probably lived in the 1st century A.D.

MANTIAS: Follower of Herophilus, renowned as a pharmacologist. Lived in the second half of the 2nd century B.C.

MILTIADES: Otherwise unknown.

MNASEAS: Methodist physician of the 1st century A.D.

MNESITHEUS: Athenian physician probably of the later part of the 4th century B.C. Among his works was one on child-rearing of which Oribasius, *Collect. med.* 54, 19 (vol. 3, p. 153 f., cf. *ibid.*, p. 682), has preserved a fragment. The passages in Soranus, pp. 102 and 118 probably refer to this work.

MOSCHION: Chiefly known as pharmacologist; probably lived at the beginning of the Christian era. He must not be confounded with Muscio, the late Latin interpreter of Soranus.

PHAEDRUS: Otherwise unknown.

POLYARCHUS: Pharmacological writer mentioned by Celsus (v, 18, 8 and VIII, 9, 1 D); probably lived before the beginning of the Christian era. See materia medica s.v. Cataplasm.

SIMON THE MAGNESIAN: Ilberg refers to Diogenes Laertius who (II, 1243) mentions "a physician, in the time of Seleucus Nicanor" by the name of Simon.

SOSTRATUS: Physician and zoologist, date unknown. Celsus (VII, prooem.) mentions him among the outstanding Alexandrian surgeons.

STRATON THE ERASISTRATEAN: Alexandrian physician of the 3rd century B.C.

THEMISON (see Introduction, p. xxvii): His work on "Chronic Diseases" was probably the first monograph devoted to this group of diseases.

THESSALUS (see Introduction, p. xxvii)

XENOPHON: Either of two physicians of this name, who lived in the 4th and 3rd centuries B.C. respectively.

ZENON THE EPICUREAN: Contemporary of Cicero.

MATERIA MEDICA

ABSINTHIUM: Recommended by the "heterodox" for pica, but rejected by Soranus because apt to cause miscarriage, 53. In abortifacients, 66, 67, 68. In suppositories in metasyncritic treatment of chronic amenorrhea and dysmenorrhea, 142. In plaster for physometra, 156.

ACACIA [According to Dioscorides I, 101 (vol. 1, p. 92 f.), it was mainly the dried juice squeezed from the fruit that was used, but also the gum.]: As astringent for upset stomach in pica, 51. Rejected by Soranus for physometra, 157. Juice injected for hemorrhage of the uterus, 163; in plasters for hemorrhage of the uterus, 163. For gonorrhea, 169. Juice for moistening tampon in prolapse of the uterus, 205.

ALMOND: As food in pica, 53. Roasted almonds in cough lozenges, 124.

ALOE: As astringent for upset stomach in pica, 51. In plaster for hemorrhage of the uterus, 163.

ALUM [Soranus, p. 51, mentions dry and moist alum. Dioscorides V, 106 (vol. 3, p. 75) and Pliny XXXV, 183 f. (vol. 9, p. 394 f.) distinguish various kinds. According to the latter, the most renowned alum came from Egypt and Melos as "liquidum spissumque." Galen, ed. Kühn, vol. 12, p. 236, writes: "The name of this medicament (*styptēria*) is taken from the astringency (*stypsis*) which it possesses to a very high degree. Although of coarse particles, the so-called lamellose alum is of somewhat finer particles than the others. Next come the round and the dice shaped. The moist alum and those kinds called *plakitis* and *plinthitis* are rather coarse." For a detailed discussion cf. Singer, p. 21 ff.; also Partington, *passim*]: Dry or moist alum as astringent for upset stomach in pica, 51. Moist alum used topically as contraceptive, 64; in contraceptive suppository, 65. In plaster to effect drying up milk of breast, 77; moist alum in ointment to dry up milk, 78. For skin ulcers of infants, 123. In plaster for hemorrhage of the uterus, 163.

AMARAKOS: Usually believed to be identical with marjoram. However, Soranus mentions oil of both marjoram and *amarakos* as ingredients of vaginal suppositories in the treatment of mole, 160.

AMULET: Contraceptive, 66. In hemorrhage of the uterus without material effect, yet psychologically helpful, 165.

ANISE: Soranus denies that anise promotes quick labor, 195.

ANTELOPE: As food in pica, 52. As food for wet nurse in later stages of nursing, 100.

ANTHERA REMEDY [Galen, ed. Kühn, vol. 12, p. 957, gives the following composition of an "*anthēra* remedy" as he found it in Soranus. "Illyrian iris, Realgar, Cyperus, ana 4 drachms, Lamellose alum, Myrrh, Saffron, Saffron dregs, ana 2 drachms" (Saffron dregs are residue after preparation of saffron ointment). The *anthēra* remedies formed a special class in the composition of which flower blossoms played a great role as the name indicates; cf. also Celsus VI, 11, 2 and *passim* (vol. 2, p. 254, footnote and *ibid.* p. xxviii) and Galen, ed. Kühn, vol. 13, p. 839.]: For application in thrush, 121.

APHRONITRE [Exact nature of aphronitre not known, probably similar to natron; cf. Galen, ed. Kühn, vol. 12, p. 212]: For sprinkling newborn infants, 83. "White aphronitre" in suppositories for physometra, 156.

APPLE: Externally as styptic remedy for upset stomach in pica, 51; baked apple as food in pica, 52. Odoriferous analeptic in labor, 70. Apple as food in hemorrhage of uterus, 164. Decoction for flux of women, 167. As food in difficult labor, 186.

ASHES: Of sea sponge or dry dregs of wine in suppositories for hemorrhage of uterus, 164. Straton uses moistened ashes in prolapse of uterus, which Soranus rejects, 204.

ASPARAGUS: "Wild" asparagus recommended as food in pica (probably *Asparagus acutifolius* and identical with Dioscorides II, 125, "rock" asparagus), 52.

ASSES' MILK: Although recommended by Hippocrates, asses' milk is rejected by Soranus in hysteria, 153.

ASSIAN STONE [According to Galen, ed. Kühn, vol. 12, p. 202, the stone came from Assus and was also called "flower of Assian rock." Pliny, XXXVI, 131 (ed. Ianus, Lipsiae 1878) relates that "in Assus of the Troad" a stone is used for coffins which consumes the bodies of the dead within 40 days, except their teeth. Dioscorides v, 124 recommends the "flower" forming on top of the stone, chiefly in treatment of wounds]: Only psychologically effective in hemorrhage of the uterus, 165.

BALSAM [*Opobalsamon,* the true balm of Mecca, the juice from *Balsamodendron gileadense*]: Used as topical contraceptive, 64.

BARLEY: Finest meal of barley as styptic for upset stomach in pica, 51; meal as styptic poultice for pains in pica, 52; porridge of barley groats as food in pica, 52. Odoriferous analeptic in labor, 70. Juice in sprinkling of newborn, 83. "Kneaded barley meal" rejected as ingredient of early baby food, 88. Juice dropped into baby's mouth in tonsillitis, 121. Powder in poultice for skin ulcerations of children, 123; "the remedy . . . of barley corn" to cicatrize skin ulcers, 123. Barley in poultice in physometra, 156. Powder in plasters for hemorrhage of the uterus, 163. Juice injected in flux of women, 167. Liquid barley gruel as food in difficult labor, 186. Cold juice given as food in prolapse of uterus by Euryphon, but rejected by Soranus, 203; barley groats for poulticing abdomen in prolapse of the uterus, 205 f.

BASS: Food for wet nurse, 99.

BAT: Soranus rejects ashes of burnt bats to stimulate the production of milk in wet nurses, 102.

BAYBERRY: In sitz baths in treatment of mole, 160. (For the "bayberry cataplasm" see under "cataplasm.")

BED BUG: Soranus rejects the use of squashed bed bugs for hysteria as recommended by most followers of other sects, 152 f. [Dioscorides II, 34 (vol. 1, p. 133): ". . . those suffering from hysterical suffocation are aroused when they smell (bed bugs)."]

BIRDS: Domestic birds as food in pica, 52. The young of domestic birds food for wet nurse, 99.

BITUMEN: To smell bitumen in hysteria rejected by Soranus, 152 f.; in wine for hysteria recommended by Mantias, 153. Fumigations

BRINE: Brine and its mixture with vinegar rejected by Soranus for drying up milk in breast, 78. Wine mixed with brine for washing newborns rejected by Soranus, 82. To be avoided in infantile exanthemata as too pungent, 122. In sitz baths etc. for mole during remissions, 160.

BUTTER: To be avoided in early baby food, 88. Not to be used for anointing gums of baby while teething, 120. In suppositories in metasyncritic treatment of chronic amenorrhea and dysmenorrhea, 142. Recommended by some ancients, but rejected by Soranus for inflammation of the uterus, 148. In vaginal suppositories for mole, 160.

CABBAGE: Ingredient for drying up clotted breasts, 78. Decoction given to hysterical patients by Hippocrates, 153.

CADMIA [Some zinc compound, possibly calamine. Dioscorides v, 74 mentions various kinds of cadmia and states that it has the power to astringe, to fill up cavities, to cleanse, etc.]: For cicatrization of skin ulcers, 123.

CALF: Calf's rennet in flux of women, 167.

CANTHARIS (Spanish fly): Euryphon uses cantharides for vaginal suppositories in retention of secundines, but Soranus objects, 197.

CAPER (*Capparis spinosa L.*): Soranus rejects capers for making the milk of wet nurses thinner, 103.

CARDAMOM: In abortifacient, 68. Rejected by Soranus in lozenge for wheezing of infants, 124.

CARROT: In sitz baths for physometra, 156.

CASSIA: In sitz baths for physometra, 156. Fumigations in retention of secundines rejected by Soranus, 197 f.

CASTOREUM: Recommended by many in hysteria, but rejected by Soranus, 152 f. Straton censured for recommending castoreum in prolapse of the uterus, 204.

CATAPLASM:

Bayberry cataplasm [Galen, ed. Kühn, vol. 13, pp. 259 and 979 gives some formulae which contained several ingredients]: For chronic amenorrhea and dysmenorrhea, 142. For physometra, 156. For mole, 160.

Cephisophon's cataplasm [Composition unknown]: In treatment of mole during remissions, 160.

Diachylon cataplasm (see Diachylon).

Mnaseas' cataplasm [Galen, ed. Kühn, vol. 13, p. 962 mentions a plaster composed by Mnaseas consisting of old olive oil, litharge, and pig's fat]: In treatment of exacerbations of mole, 160.

Polyarchus' cataplasm [According to Celsus v, 18, 8 (vol. 2, p. 21), it contains "square rush, cardamon, frankincense soot, amomum, wax and liquid resin in equal quantities." Galen, ed. Kühn, vol. 13, p. 184 f. gives a more complicated formula]: For physometra, 156. For mole during remissions, 160.

Seed cataplasm [Galen, ed. Kühn, vol. 13, p. 261 gives two formulae containing numerous ingredients]: For chronic amenorrhea and dysmenorrhea, 142. For physometra, 156. For mole, 160.

CEDAR RESIN: As local contraceptive, 64. Rejected by Soranus for hysteria, 152 f. Soranus denies that cedar resin promotes quick birth, 195.

CELERY: For drying up breasts in which clotting has set in (cf. Dioscorides III, 64), 78. Soranus rejects seed in draughts for retention of secundines, 197 f.

CENTAURY: Dioscorides III, 6 and 7, as well as Galen, ed. Kühn, vol. 12, p. 19 ff. distinguish between a large centaury (*Centaurea salonitana*) and a small centaury (feverwort). Soranus probably refers to the former in metasyncritic treatment of mole, 160.

CERATE: With various ingredients for pica, 51. Cerate containing oil from unripe olives and myrtle as ointment on pregnant abdomen, 57. Containing myrtle oil and white lead as topical contraceptive, 64. Wax salve in after treatment of inflamed breast, 77. Moist wax salve with white of egg for inflamed sores of children, 123. Cerates in after treatment of dysmenorrhea and amenorrhea, 141; wax for emollient suppository in amenorrhea and dysmenorrhea, 141. Wax salves in hysteria, 152. Wax salve added to a plaster for physometra, 156. Cerates with various ingredients for exacerbations in mole, 160. With various ingredients for hemorrhage of the uterus, 163. Cerates for gonorrhea, 169.

CEREAL FOOD: Dangers of premature feeding of infants with cereals, 117; selection of cereal food from 6 months on, 117; cereal food and weaning, 118. Food "of the cereal type" advised in early stage of pregnancy, 46.

CHALCITES [A mineral found in Cyprus of unknown composition but probably containing copper and sulphur; cf. Partington, p. 364 and Singer, p. 14. Dioscorides v, 99 (vol. 3, p. 70) especially mentions its use in hemorrhage of the uterus]: In vaginal suppositories for hemorrhage of the uterus, 164.

CHASTE TREE (*Vitex agnus-castus*): One drachm of the seed in water for gonorrhea, 169.

CHEESE: To be avoided in atony of the uterus, 172.

CHICKEN FAT: For softening baby's gums before teething, 120. In suppository for dysmenorrhea, 140. In vaginal suppositories for mole, 160.

CIMOLIAN EARTH [Cf. p. 64, footnote 124 and Dioscorides v, 156]: In contraceptive suppository, 64.

CORIANDER: In diagnosis of fertility, 33. To suppress milk, 77.

COW PARSNIP (*Heracleum sphondylium*): Abortifacient, 65.

CRAY FISH [*Karabos;* this, as discussed by Aristotle (De partibus animalium IV, 8, and "Hist. animal." IV, 2 and VIII, 2; 590 b 10 ff.), is usually identified with the spiny lobster, *Palinurus vulgaris*]: Food in pica, 52.

CUCUMBER (see also Melon): Seed used with water by the "heterodox" for pica, 53. As odoriferous analeptic in labor, 70; Soranus denies that the "fruit of the wild cucumber" promotes quick birth, 195.

CUMMIN: Externally for drying up milk in breasts, 78. Rejected as pungent by Soranus in treatment of navel stump, 84. Roasted cummin rejected for poultice in tonsillitis because causing congestion of the head, 121. Rejected by Soranus in lozenges for wheezing of infants, 124. In suppositories in metasyncritic treatment of chronic amenorrhea and dysmenorrhea, 142.

CYATH: The Attic *kyathos* was about $1/12$ of a pint. Its weight, according to Pliny XXI, 185, was 10 drachms.

CYCLAMEN: Root in suppository for physometra, 156.

CYPERUS: Externally for drying up milk, 78. For thrush, 121.

CYRENAIC BALM [The juice obtained from silphium, probably the name for various plants, laserwort among others]: In abortifacients, 65.

DATE: Dry dates in plaster for upset stomach in pica [Dioscorides I, 109 (vol. 1, 102) says of dry dates that they help those spitting blood, suffering from the stomach, etc.], 51. Tender dates in antiphlogistic application to breasts, 77. For poulticing skin ulcers of infants, 123. Rejects Theban dates for plasters in physometra, 157. In plasters for hemorrhage of the uterus, 163, 164. Decoction of Theban dates for flux of women, 167. Externally for gonorrhea, 169. For poulticing abdomen in prolapse of the uterus, 205; in plasters for chronically prolapsed uterus, 206. Juicy Dates [*patētos phoinix;* Pliny XIII, 45 (vol. 4, p. 125), speaking of the "pateta," writes that this class of dates "has too copious a supply of juice, and the excess of liquor of the fruit itself bursts open even while on the parent tree, looking like dates that have been trodden on"]: In suppositories for dysmenorrhea and amenorrhea, 140.

DATE SALVE: See p. 196 and footnote 55.

DAUCUS: Cretan daucus (probably *Athamanta cretensis*) in sitz baths for physometra, 156.

DEER (see also Hartshorn): Marrow or brain in vaginal suppositories for mole, 160. Rennet for flux of women, 167.

DIACHYLON [On the meaning of diachylon see p. 123, footnote 81]: Diachylon remedy for ulcerations of infants, 123. Diachylon suppository in after treatment of amenorrhea and dysmenorrhea, 141. Diachylon cataplasm in exacerbation of mole, 160.

DILL: In food in dysmenorrhea, 138.

DIOSPOLIS REMEDY [According to Galen, ed. Kühn, vol. 6, p. 265, the remedy consisted of cummin, pepper, rue, and natron. Because of the latter ingredient it seems likely that the remedy was named after Diospolis, a city of Egypt]: For physometra, 157.

DITTANY: Externally in metasyncritic treatment of mole, 160. Soranus denies its effectiveness for quick birth, 195. Euryphon uses potion, Straton fomentation for retention of secundines, but Soranus disapproves, 197 f.

DUCK: Wild duck as food in pica, 52.

EGG: Soft boiled as food in pica, 50, 52. For wet nurse, 99; "eggs that can be sipped" for wet nurse when her milk has become too thin, 103. "Egg that can be sipped" as baby food, 117. White of egg in ointment for inflamed sores of infants, 123; "the remedy of eggs" applied to skin ulcers of infants to promote cicatrization, 123. Yolk diluted with rose oil on bregma in siriasis, 125. In vaginal application in dysmenorrhea, 137; "eggs that can be sipped" as food in dysmenorrhea, 138; yolk of egg in vaginal suppository for dysmenorrhea, 140. Soft boiled egg as food in hemorrhage of the uterus, 164. White of eggs instilled if closed uterus causes difficult labor, 185.

ENDIVE [According to Dioscorides II, 132, *seris* exists in a wild and two cultivated forms, all of which are "styptic, cooling and good for the stomach" (vol. 1, p. 204, 5)]: Raw or cooked as food in pica, 52. In poultice for extensive ulcerations of skin in children, 123. Juice injected in hemorrhage of the uterus, 163; in plasters for hemorrhage of the uterus, 163; as food in hemorrhage of the uterus, 164.

FAR [Probably some kind of spelt. Aretaeus (Adams' translation, p. 428) in his chapter on the "Cure of Bringing up Blood" writes: "and the Tuscan *far* is a very excellent thing, being thick, viscid, and glutinous when given along with the milk"]: As porridge for wet nurse when her milk is too thin, 103.

FAT: Goose fat in suppositories before parturition, 57. Fat for softening gums before teething, 120. Fresh warm pork fat with bread as poultice for dysmenorrhea, 139; fresh goose or chicken fat in suppository for dysmenorrhea, 140; ox fat and fat of any kind in suppositories for amenorrhea and dysmenorrhea, 141. In suppositories for hysteria, 151. Goose fat and chicken fat in vaginal suppositories in mole, 160.

FENUGREEK [Generally recognized as *Trigonella foenum-graecum L.*]: In sitz bath for relaxation of genitals before parturition, 57. In abortifacients, 66. In antiphlogistic poultice for breast, 77; decoction as fomentation for breast, 77. Juice for mitigating effect of salt in sprinkling newborn, 83. For poultices in teething, 120. Decoction for bathing inflamed sores of infants, 123. Decoction for dysmenorrhea, 137; in various poultices for dysmenorrhea, 139; juice in suppository together with hot decoction externally for amenorrhea and dysmenorrhea, 140. In suppositories for hysteria, 151. Decoction instilled if closure of orifice of uterus causes difficult labor, 185; for poultice in difficult labor, 185. Juice of boiled fenugreek for bathing inveterate prolapsed uterus, 206.

FIG: Flesh of dried figs in contraceptive suppository, 65. Dried for drying up milk in breast, 78. Dried as rubefacient for physometra, 156; boiled for poulticing in physometra, 156; in plaster for physometra, 156; rich figs in suppositories for physometra, 156. Dried as rubefacient in mole during remissions, 160; flesh of dried rich figs in vaginal suppositories for mole, 160.

FISH: Fish which are not greasy as food in early pregnancy, 47. Fishes living among rocks as food for wet nurse, 99; tender fish food for wet nurse during 2nd and 3rd week, 99. Delicate fish as bland food in metasyncritic treatment of chronic amenorrhea and dysmenorrhea, 142.

FLEABANE [Both Dioscorides III, 121 and Galen, ed. Kühn, vol. 12, p. 35, recommend fleabane as an emmenagogue]: "The so-called thin-leaved" fleabane (probably *Inula graveolens*) in vaginal suppositories for metasyncritic treatment of chronic amenorrhea and dysmenorrhea, 142.

FLEAWORT: For drying up milk in breast, 77. Juice injected for hemorrhage of the uterus, 163; in plasters for hemorrhage of the uterus, 163.

FLOCK: Burnt flock for hysteria rejected by Soranus, 152 f.

FOWL: As food in pica, 50, 52. As food for wet nurse, 100. In late stage of metasyncritic treatment of amenorrhea and dysmenorrhea, 142. Roasted as food in gonorrhea, 169.

FRANCOLIN: As food in pica, 52. Breast as food in hemorrhage of the uterus, 164.

FRANKINCENSE: Frankincense and bark of the frankincense tree for thrush, 122. Pulverized in suppositories for hemorrhage of the uterus, 164.

GALBANUM [Mentioned as a spice in Exodus 30, 34; "the resinous juice of all-heal, *Ferula galbaniflua*" (Liddell and Scott)]: Topically with wine as contraceptive, 64. In suppositories for physometra, 156. Rejected by Soranus for fumigations in retention of secundines, 197 f.

GARLIC [*Skorodon* and *skordon;* the two terms are used synonymously and refer to *Allium sativum L.* On this and related plants, cf. Kurt Heyser, Die Alliumarten als Arzneimittel im Gebrauch der abendländischen Medizin, *Kyklos* 1928, 1, pp. 64–102]: Used by others in fertility test, 33. Forbidden, as pungent, to newly pregnant women, 47. Makes milk of wet nurse pungent, 99.

GARLIC GERMANDER (*Teucrium scordium*): Externally in metasyncritic treatment of mole, 160; Soranus rejects its use for steaming in same disease, 161.

GERMANDER: Externally in metasyncritic treatment of mole, 160.

GINGER [Probably the rhizome of *Zingiber officinale*]: In contraceptive suppository, 65.

GOAT'S MARJORAM [According to Liddell and Scott, goat's marjoram is *Thymus teucrioides*]: Cretan goat's marjoram recommended by the "heterodox" in pica, 53.

GOOSE FAT: For emollient suppository before parturition, 57. In suppository for dysmenorrhea, 140. In suppositories for mole, 160.

GRAPES: Preserved, as food in pica, 53.

GRAPESTONES: Ground in potion for flux of women, 167.

GROUND GRAIN: For poulticing in painful pica, 52. Lukewarm in amenorrhea and dysmenorrhea, 136. For poulticing in physometra, 156. Warm ground grain for difficult labor, 185.

GUM [*Kommi;* according to Dioscorides I, 101, it is obtained from acacia]: In contraceptive suppository, 65.

GUM LADANUM ["Ladanum or ledanum was the resinous secretion of the leaves and flowers of several varieties of Cistus" (H. E. Sigerist, Laudanum in the Works of Paracelsus, *Bull. Hist. Med.* 1941, vol. 9, p. 532). According to Dioscorides I, 97 (vol. 1, p. 88) ladanum, applied with wine, makes wound scars better looking.]: "The remedy of gum ladanum" for ulcers of infants to promote cicatrization, 123.

HAIR: Against those recommending smell of burnt hair for hysteria, 152 f. Rejects fumigation with human hair in retention of secundines, 197 f. Rejects application of hairy bags in prolapse of the uterus, 203.

HALIKAKABON [Dioscorides IV, 71 and 72 distinguishes two plants of this name. The plant here referred to is possibly the *strychnon hypnōtikon* of which Dioscorides IV, 72, Theophrastus IX, XI, 5, and Galen, ed. Kühn, vol. 12, p. 145, say that the bark of its root

dysmenorrhea, 139; in suppositories for dysmenorrhea, 140; in suppositories for metasyncritic treatment of chronic amenorrhea and dysmenorrhea, 142. Honey water in hysterical paroxysm, 151. In poultice and suppositories for physometra, 156. In vaginal suppositories for mole, 160. In vaginal suppositories and fomentations in retention of secundines rejected by Soranus, 197 f.

HONEY WINE [According to Dioscorides v, 8 it was usually prepared in the proportion of 1 part honey to 2 parts of wine.]: As beverage for the wet nurse after 40 days, 100. Crumbs of bread softened in honey wine for older babies, 117. Draughts of honey wine rejected in mole, 161.

HOREHOUND: In sitz baths for physometra, 156. Decoction for sitz baths etc. for mole, 160; steaming with the leaves for mole rejected by Soranus, 161. Fumigations with horehound in retention of secundines rejected by Soranus, 197 f.

HOUSELEEK [Dioscorides IV, 88–90 distinguishes 3 kinds of *aeizōon*, one of which is *Sempervivum arboreum L.*, while the others are doubtful]: For poulticing extensive skin ulcerations in infants, 123.

HYDROMEL: Used by the "heterdox" for pica, 53. For antiphlogistic poultice for breast, 77. Early baby food, 88; crumbs of bread softened in hydromel for older babies, 117. Bread kneaded in warm hydromel as poultice for amenorrhea and dysmenorrhea, 136. For poulticing in difficult labor, 185; with water for enema in difficult labor, 186.

HYPOCIST: As astringent for upset stomach in pica, 51. Juice injected in persistent hemorrhage of the uterus, 163. In plasters for hemorrhage of the uterus, 163. For gonorrhea, 169. Juice diluted in wine for moistening tampon in prolapse of the uterus, 205.

HYSSOP [It is doubtful whether the hyssop of the ancients was identical with *Hyssopus officinalis*. Liddell and Scott identify it with *Origanum hirtum*.]: Recommmended in pica by the "heterodox," 53. In suppositories in metasyncritic treatment of chronic amenorrhea and dysmenorrhea, 142. For poultice, plaster, sitz bath, suppositories in physometra, 156. Decoction in sitz baths, etc. and in suppository for mole during remissions, 160.

IRIS: Oil for abortifacient, 66. With honey or dry for thrush, 122. In suppositories for physometra, 156. Oil for irrigation in soft swelling of the uterus, 158. Oil in suppositories in mole, 160. Euryphon recommends Illyrian iris in suppositories for retention of secundines, but Soranus rejects it, 197 f. (According to Dioscorides I, 1, Illyrian and Macedonian irises are superior to others.)

IVY: Externally for drying up milk in breast, 78.

KID: As food in pica, 52. Meat as food for wet nurse, 100; meat for wet nurses whose milk is too thin, 103.

KNOTGRASS: Juice injected for hemorrhage of the uterus, 163; plaster for hemorrhage of the uterus, 163.

LAMB: Rennet in flux of women, 167.

LAMP WICKS: Soranus rejects use of extinguished lamp wicks in hysteria, 152.

LEAD: For treatment of navel stump, 114. Leaden plate beneath the loins at night time for gonorrhea, 169. Large piece appended by Mantias to placenta for extraction, but rejected by Soranus, 197 f.

LEEK: Rejected as pungent for newly pregnant woman, 47. Rejected for wet nurse, 99.

LEMON [The *kitrion* is some kind of citrous fruit]: Odoriferous analeptic for labor, 70.

LENTILS: In astringent poultices for thrush, 121. Warm decoction for skin affections of children, 122; husked and boiled with honey for cleansing infants' sores, 123. Decoction for sitz baths or injection in hemorrhage of the uterus, 162 f. With oxymel for poulticing abdomen in prolapse of the uterus, 206.

LICORICE: Juice in cough lozenges, 124.

LILY [Soranus calls the oil of lilies *elaion Sousinon,* which corresponds with Dioscorides' statement, III, 102 (vol. 2, p. 113, 1–2) that an ointment is prepared from lilies "which some people call Sousinon."]: Oil in after treatment of amenorrhea and dysmenorrhea, 141; oil in suppositories for metasyncritic treatment of chronic amenorrhea and dysmenorrhea, 142. Oil in suppositories for hysteria, 151. Oil in suppositories for mole, 160. Oil for uterine injections in atony of the uterus, 172. Oil for fomentations in retention of secundines rejected by Soranus, 197 f.

LINSEED: In sitz baths to relax genitals before parturition, 57. For abortifacients, 66. For antiphlogistic poultice for breast, 77; decoction for fomentation of breast, 77. For poultices in teething, 120; decoction for bathing inflamed sores of infants, 123. In cough lozenges, 124. For poultice in amenorrhea and dysmenorrhea, 136; decoction for dysmenorrhea, 137; for poultice in dysmenorrhea, 139; in suppository together with hot decoction externally for amenorrhea and dysmenorrhea, 140. Decoction instilled if closed orifice of uterus causes difficult labor, 185; for poultice in difficult labor, 185. Juice for bathing inveterate prolapsed uterus, 206.

LITHARGE: For anointing infants' parts squeezed during delivery, 84. For anointing skin ulcers of infants, 123; for "filling up" the cavities of sores in infants, 123.

LOTUS [Galen, ed. Kühn, vol. 12, p. 65, says of the lotus tree (possibly the nettle tree) that the filings of its wood are good for "female flux, dysentery, and abdominal conditions."]: Infusion of sawdust in potion for flux of women, 167.

LUPINES: Meal of lupines for abortifacient, 67; likewise bitter lupines, 67 f. (Bitter lupines are probably those that have not been macerated in water; cf. Dioscorides II, 109).

MAGNET: Only psychologically effective in hemorrhage of the uterus, 165.

MALABATHRON (Possibly *Cinnamomum Tamala*): Oil in suppositories for mole, 160.

MALLOW [Dioscorides II, 118 mentions the garden mallow and the wild mallow, but the differential identification of the two seems uncertain. Liddell and Scott suggest *Lavatera arborea* for the garden variety.]: Decoction for sitz bath for relaxing genitals before parturition, 57. In abortifacients, 66. Decoction for fomentation of breast, 77. Juice for mitigating effect of salt for sprinkling newborn, 83. Decoction of roots of the wild mallow for bathing inflamed sores of infants, 123. Decoction of "mallow cultivated or even wild" for dysmenorrhea, 137; roots of wild mallow in poultice for dysmenorrhea, 139; decoction in poultice for dysmenorrhea, 139; in suppository together with hot decoction of "mallow, either cultivated or wild" externally for amenorrhea and

analeptic for labor, 70. "The skin surrounding the flesh of a melon" for siriasis, 125. As food in difficult labor, 186.

MILK: For breast feeding, 88 ff. Goat's milk in early baby food, 89; crumbs of bread softened in milk for older babies, 117. Asses' milk (q.v.), 153. To mitigate very irritant suppository for physometra, 156. To be avoided in atony of the uterus, 172. Milk pills, 102.

MILLET: For loose bowels of infants suffering from skin troubles, 124.

MINT REMEDY (composition unknown): For physometra, 157.

MULES: Soranus rejects the alleged contraceptive effect of amulets of mule's uterus and of dirt in mules' ears, 66.

MUSSELS: As food in pica, 52.

MUSTARD [For the indications for and preparation of the mustard plaster see Oribasius, *Collect. med.* 10, 13 (vol. 2, p. 410 ff.)]: "The mustard remedy" (composition uncertain) recommended for pica by the "heterodox," 53. As rubefacient in metasyncritic treatment of chronic amenorrhea and dysmenorrhea, 142. Mustard plasters in metasyncritic treatment of chronic hysteria, 152. As rubefacient for physometra, 156. As rubefacient for mole during remissions, 160. Mustard plaster for flux of women, 168. Mustard plaster in chronically prolapsing uterus, 206.

MYRRH: In abortifacients, 65, 68. For thrush, 122. Fumigations rejected for mole, 161. In draughts for retention of secundines rejected by Soranus, 197 f.

MYRTLE: Oil as astringent for upset stomach in pica, 51. Oil in cerate for the pregnant abdomen, 57. Oil in cerate used topically as contraceptive, 64. In abortifacients, 65, 67, 68. For sprinkling newborn; rejected by Soranus as astringent but not cleansing, 82 f.; leaves put by some into cradle to give it sweet smell, 87. Warm decoction in skin affection of children, 122; oil in ointment for skin ulcers of infants, 123. Decoction for sitz bath or vaginal injection for hemorrhage of the uterus, 162 f.; leaves or oil in plasters for hemorrhage of the uterus, 163. Decoction as sitz bath in gonorrhea, 169; externally in gonorrhea, 169. Decoction as sitz bath in prolapse of the uterus, 205; decoction of berries externally for hemorrhage of uterus, 162; berries for stuffing meat in hemorrhage of uterus, 164. Berries in potion for flux of women, 167.

NARCISSUS: Oil for uterine injections in atony of the uterus, 172.

NARD: Oil as astringent for upset stomach in pica, 51; infusion of Syrian nard recommended by the "heterodox" in pica, 53. Suppositories recommended by physicians of other sects for hysteria, 152. For sitz bath in physometra, 156. Fomentations for retention of secundines rejected by Soranus, 197 f.

NATRON [A native sodium carbonate containing various impurities (cf. F. W. Gibbs, On "Nitre" and "Natron," *Annals of Science,* 1938, vol. 3, pp. 213–16). Widely used as a detergent; cf. Plato, *Timaeus,* 60 D.]: In contraceptive suppository, 65. For sprinkling newborn infants, 83. For gentle cleansing of infants' skin irritations, 123. Locally in metasyncritic treatment of chronic amenorrhea and dysmenorrhea, 142; for suppositories in metasyncritic treatment of chronic amenorrhea and dysmenorrhea, 142. Externally and in suppositories for physometra, 156. Sprinkled for mole, 160. In suppositories in after treatment of chronically prolapsing uterus, but not while the uterus is still prolapsed, 206.

NAVELWORT [Probably *Cotyledon umbilicus L.* although Dioscorides IV, 92 also mentions another kind of *Kotylēdōn.*]: For poulticing extensive skin ulcerations in infants, 123.

NETTLE [Cf. Dioscorides IV, 93 (vol. 2, p. 252, 6 ff.)]: Seed in lozenges for wheezing of infants rejected by Soranus, 124.

NIGHTSHADE (probably black nightshade, *Solanum nigrum L.*): Juice in treatment of siriasis, 125 [likewise recommended by Dioscorides IV, 70]. Juice recommended by Themison, but rejected by Soranus for febrile inflammation of the uterus, 148. Juice injected for hemorrhage of the uterus, 163; in plasters for hemorrhage of the uterus, 163.

NOSESMART (a cress, but identification with *Lepidium sativum* doubtful): Used by various predecessors of Soranus in diagnosis of fertility, 33. Rejected in baby food, 88. Rejected in potion for mole, 161.

OAK: Leaves in decoction for sitz baths or juice for injection in hemorrhage of the uterus, 162 f.

OAK GALL (see also *omphakitis* oak gall): As astringent for upset stomach in pica, 51. In contraceptive suppository, 65 f. For sprinkling newborn, yet rejected by Soranus as astringent but not

cleansing, 82 f. For thrush, 122. For vaginal suppositories for hemorrhage of the uterus, 164.

OBOL: 1/6 of a drachm; cf. Pliny XXI, 185.

OLIVE [On oil and olives see the note in Bussemaker et Daremberg, *Oeuvres d'Oribase,* vol. 1, p. 609. The oil from unripe olives is the *omphacium* of Pliny XII, 130 and the *omphakinon* of Dioscorides I, 30, 1.]: Pickled in brine as food in pica, 52.

OLIVE OIL: Warm, for suppositories in menarche, 22. Freshly extracted from unripe olives as ointment in early pregnancy, 46. From freshly ground, unripe olives for embrocations over abdomen in severe pica, 51. From unripe olives in cerate for the pregnant abdomen, 57; for injections before parturition, 57. Old olive oil locally as contraceptive, 64. Warm oil and old olive oil as abortifacients, 66. Warm upon abdomen and genitals in preparation for labor, 72 f.; for anointing midwife's hands, 72 f. In antiphlogistic poultice of breast, 77. To mitigate effect of salt used for sprinkling newborn, 83. For eyes of newborn as a protective measure, 83. For dressing umbilical stump, 84. For cleansing mouth of the newborn, 104. For anointing infants, 104, 107, 108. On wool externally and injected into ear in teething, 120. Old oil with salt, used by nurses in rubbing inflamed tonsils, but rejected by Soranus, 121. In ointment for itching of infant, 122; with water for bathing inflamed sores of infants, 123. Warm and applied externally for amenorrhea and dysmenorrhea, 136; warm and mixed with water for dysmenorrhea as sitz bath, or with egg and various decoctions vaginally, 137; in gruel for food in dysmenorrhea, 138; in poultice for dysmenorrhea, 139; warm enema for dysmenorrhea, 139; warm in suppositories for amenorrhea and dysmenorrhea, 140; with water used warm for external application of heat in dysmenorrhea, 140; for anointing abdomen in dysmenorrhea, 140; in suppositories and bath in after treatment of amenorrhea and dysmenorrhea, 141; for suppositories in metasyncritic treatment of chronic amenorrhea and dysmenorrhea, 142. As a relaxing warm enema and injected in inflammation of the uterus, 147; with a decoction of rue and greasy wool recommended by some ancients, but rejected by Soranus for inflammation of the uterus, 148. On lower abdomen in hysterical

facient potion, 65. For abdominal poultices in prolapse of the uterus, 206.

OYSTERS: As food in pica, 52.

PANAX [Hippocrates, ed. Littré, vol. 8, p. 387 mentions *panakes* as remedy for displacement of the uterus, and Littré interprets it as *Echinophora tenuifolia*. Dioscorides III, 48 says of the *panakes Hērakleion* that the balm (*opopanax*) was gathered from it and that its "root, if scraped and applied to the uterus, expells the fetus" (vol. 2, p. 63, 11).]: Root in contraceptive suppository, 64. Balm in abortifacients, 65, 66. Balm used by "the ancients" as hemagogue in dysmenorrhea, but rejected by Soranus, 139.

PAPYRUS: For making the "black remedy" (q.v.).

PARSLEY: Oil with bread recommended by some ancients in inflammation of the uterus, but rejected by Soranus, 148.

PARSNIP [Dioscorides II, 113 (vol. 1, p. 188) says of the "well-known *sisaron*" that its boiled root "is good for the stomach, moves the urine and stimulates the appetite." According to Berendes, p. 215, the identification of *sisaron* as parsnip is uncertain.]: As food in pica, 52.

PARTRIDGE: As food in pica, 52. Breast as food in hemorrhage of the uterus, 164.

PEARS: As food in pica, 53. Boiled as food in hemorrhage of the uterus, 164.

PELLITORY: Used by the ancients as a hemagogue, but rejected by Soranus, 139.

PENNYROYAL: As odoriferous analeptic in labor, 70 (Dioscorides III, 31 mentions it as an analeptic). In sitz bath and suppository in physometra, 156. Decoction in sitz baths, etc. for mole during remissions, 160; rejected for steaming and in potions for mole, 161.

PEPPER (white and black pepper are both derived from *Piper nigrum*, but distinguished by the process of drying): Seed of white pepper in abortifacient, 65. In lozenges for wheezing of infants, 124. In suppositories in metasyncritic treatment of chronic amenorrhea and dysmenorrhea, 142.

PEPPERMINT: For drying up breasts in which clotting has set in, 78 (similarly Dioscorides III, 34).

PERDIKION (probably *Polygonum maritimum*): Juice recommended by Themison in febrile inflammation of the uterus, but rejected by Soranus, 148. Juice for injections in hemorrhage of the uterus, 163; in plasters in hemorrhage of the uterus, 163.

PIG: Meat of tender pigs as food in pica, 52; meat of suckling pigs food for wet nurse, 100; pork for wet nurse in later stages of nursing, 100; feet, snouts, and ears for wet nurses whose milk is too thin, 103. Fat in poultice for dysmenorrhea, 139; fresh pork for diet in metasyncritic treatment of amenorrhea and dysmenorrhea, 142. Ankle bone, burned and ground, popularly used as powder on umbilical stump, 114.

PIGEON: As food in pica, 52. (The young of) food for wet nurse, 99.

PINE BARK [Fumigations with pine bark are recommended by Hippocrates, ed. Littré, vol. 8, p. 80, 19 in difficult labor.]: In contraceptive suppository, 64. For flux of women, 167.

PINE CONE [Galen, ed. Kühn, vol. 6, p. 591 writes: "The fruit of the pine has good and thick juices and is nourishing although not easy to digest"; cf. also Dioscorides I, 69. It is not quite clear to what kind of pine cones Soranus refers.]: As diet for wet nurses with thin milk, 103. Small pine cones for cough lozenges, 124.

PINE SEED [Dioscorides I, 69 (vol. 1, p. 66, 1): "helpful in cough and diseases of the chest."]: In cough lozenges, 124.

PITCH: For preparing suppositories for hemorrhage of the uterus (a sea sponge is soaked in the pitch and then burnt to cinders), 164; plaster locally in metasyncritic treatment of chronic amenorrhea and dysmenorrhea, 142. Plaster to effect metasyncrisis in hysteria, 152; burning of pitch rejected for hysteria, 152 f. Plaster for chronic physometra, 156. Plaster for mole, 160. Plasters to effect metasyncrisis in flux of women, 168.

PLANTAIN [According to Dioscorides II, 126 (vol. 1, p. 199, 5), the leaves have "styptic and drying power."]: As food in pica, 52. For astringent remedy in thrush, 122. In poultice for skin ulcers in infants, 123. Juice injected for infantile diarrhea, 125. Juice injected for hemorrhage of the uterus, 163; in plasters for hemorrhage of the uterus, 163; as food in hemorrhage of the uterus, 164.

POMEGRANATE [For the eating of stones of pomegranate, cf. Hippocrates, ed. Littré, vol. 6, p. 264 and Dioscorides I, 110, both of whom ascribe a constipating action to them.]: Peel as astringent for upset stomach in pica, 51; stones for pica, 52. Peel and rind in contraceptive suppositories, 64 f. Peel as astringent poultice for severe thrush, 121; juice for thrush, 122. Warm decoction of peel for skin affections of children, 123. Peel rejected by Soranus for physometra, 157. Decoction of peel for sitz baths or injection in hemorrhage of the uterus, 162 f. Peel for flux of women, 167. Diocles uses peeled pomegranates dipped in vinegar in prolapse of the uterus, but Soranus objects, 203; decoction of peel as sitz bath in prolapse of the uterus, 205; peel for poulticing abdomen in prolapse of the uterus, 206.

POPPY: Rejected in baby food, 118.

POPPYHEADS: In mouth remedy for thrush, 122.

PORK (see under Pig)

PORRIDGE (see also individual cereals, etc.): As food in early pica, 50. Food for wet nurse, 99. "Very moist" as baby food, 117.

PRESERVED MEAT OR FISH (meat or fish were preserved by salting, drying, pickling, or smoking): Rejected as pungent for newly pregnant woman, 47. Recommended by the "heterodox" for pica, 53. Rejected by Soranus for wet nurse since it makes milk pungent, 99; should not be given to wet nurse in cases of too thick milk as followers of Moschion advise, 103. Small amount in metasyncritic treatment of chronic amenorrhea and dysmenorrhea, 141.

"All preserved food" forbidden to wet nurse since it makes the milk pungent, 99.

PULSE: Rejected for wet nurse since it makes milk pungent, 99.

PUMICE STONE: Externally for drying up milk in breast, 78.

PUMPKIN: Grated for siriasis (similarly recommended by Dioscorides II, 134), 125.

PURPLE FISH (probably any mollusc belonging to any of the species of *Murex* and *Purpura*): As food in pica, 52.

PURSE TASSELS (*Muscari comosum*): Powdered bulbs upon umbilical stump (cf. above p. 114, footnote 67), 114.

PURSLANE: As food in pica, 52; recommended by the "heterodox" as infusion, decoction or food for pica, 53. In application to dry up milk in breast, 77. In poultice for skin ulcers of infants, 123. For plasters in hemorrhage of the uterus, 163.

PYRITE ["Pyrite stone" (*Lithos pyrites*) probably FeS_2 or Cu FeS_2,

skin ulcers of infants, 123. Oil for siriasis, 125. Oil with other ingredients for suppositories in inflammation of the uterus rejected by Soranus, 148. Decoction for sitz baths or vaginal injection in hemorrhage of the uterus, 162 f.; as cerate in hemorrhage of the uterus, 163; oil for plaster in hemorrhage of the uterus, 163. Decoction for sitz bath in gonorrhea, 169; oil as unguent in chronic gonorrhea, 170. Oil for uterine injections in atony of the uterus, 172. Soranus rejects fomentations with oil in retention of secundines, 197 f. Oil in water recommended by Themison for febrile inflammation of the uterus, but rejected by Soranus, 148.

RUE: Used by others in fertility test, 33. Asclepiades on its penetrating quality, 34. Seed in abortifacient, 65. Juice and leaves in abortifacients, 66, 68. With honey for suppository in metasyncritic treatment of chronic amenorrhea and dysmenorrhea, 142. Decoction with oil and dirty wool recommended by the ancients in inflammation of the uterus, but rejected by Soranus, 148. For poulticing and suppositories in physometra, 156. Seed in potion for gonorrhea, 169.

SAFFRON [For the medical history of saffron cf. Maria Tscholakowa, "Zur Geschichte der medizinischen Verwendung des Safran (Crocus sativus)," *Kyklos,* 1929, vol. 2, pp. 179–190.]: As styptic for upset stomach in pica, 51. In ointment for breast to dry up milk, 78. For thrush, 122. Fumigations rejected for mole, 161.

SALT [Dioscorides v, 109 (vol. 3, p. 80) ascribes to salt styptic as well as cleansing properties.]: "Fine and powdery salt" for sprinkling the newborn, 83. Rejected for rubbing tonsils in tonsillitis, 121. In gruel used for food in dysmenorrhea, 138; locally in metasyncritic treatment of chronic amenorrhea and dysmenorrhea, 142; for suppositories in metasyncritic treatment of chronic amenorrhea and dysmenorrhea, 142. Sprinkled in mole, 160. In suppositories for after treatment of chronically prolapsing uterus, but not while still prolapsed, 206.

SALVIA: Externally for mole during intervals, 160. Internally by Euryphon and Dion to expell secundines; rejected by Soranus, 197 f.

SAMIAN EARTH [Galen, ed. Kühn, vol. 12, p. 178 f. writes of the Samian earth: "It need not even be washed. Of its two kinds we prefer to

dysmenorrhea, 138. As food in hemorrhage of the uterus, 164. Juice injected for flux of women, 167.

SPIKENARD (see Nard)

SQUIRTING CUCUMBER: Used by the ancients as a hemagogue, but rejected by Soranus, 139.

STORAX: Rejected by Soranus for hysteria, 152 f. Rejected for mole, 161.

SUMACH [Tanning sumach, *Rhus coriaria,* described by Dioscorides I, 108, who states that its fruit is eaten.]: Tanning sumach in contraceptive suppository, 64. Decoction of tanning sumach for sitz baths or vaginal injection in hemorrhage of the uterus, 162 f.; as food in hemorrhage of the uterus, 164.

SWEET BAY: In abortifacient, 68. Leaves put by some into cradle to give it sweet smell, 87. Sweet bay or its fruit for sitz baths in physometra, 156. Decoction for sitz baths, etc. in mole during remissions, 160. Soranus denies that sweet bay promotes quick birth, 195.

SYRIAN UNGUENT (composition unknown; cf. above, p. 67 footnote 130): In abortifacient injection, 67.

TAMARISK [Dioscorides I, 87 (vol. 1, p. 82) says of the cultivated tamarisk (*T. articulata*): "It bears a fruit similar to oak galls, uneven, astringent as to its taste, suitable (instead of oak galls) for remedies for the eye and the mouth . . ."]: Fruit for thrush, 121.

THRUSH: As food in pica, 52. Recommended for wet nurse, 99.

TRAGACANTH [Dioscorides III, 20, recommends cough lozenges made of the gum with honey.]: In cough lozenges, 124.

TRAGOS [The name *tragos* is used for a variety of different substances. From the context it would appear that it means some kind of spelt (see Dioscorides II, 93, Galen, ed. Kühn, vol. 6, pp. 517 and 519). However, Dioscorides IV, 51 (vol. 2, p. 207) says of the plant *tragos* (probably *Ephedra distachya L.*) that its fruit drunk in wine "helps those suffering in the belly and women suffering from flux."]: Injection of juice in painful female flux, 167.

TRIBULUS [The name is used for a variety of plants. Dioscorides IV, 15 distinguishes 2 kinds which have been identified as *Tribulus terrestris* and *Trapa natans* respectively. Since he recommends both for inflammations (cf. vol. 2, p. 181, 8 f.), they might be identical with Soranus' "green (or fresh) tribulus."]: Green tribulus externally for drying up milk in breast, 78.

TRUMPET SHELL [Cf. D'Arcy Wentworth Thompson's footnote 7 to Aristotle's "Hist. animal." 528 a 10 (Aristotle, *Oxford transl.*).]: Recommended as food in pica, 52.

TURPENTINE: For suppository in obstinate constipation of infants, 124. For suppository in after treatment of amenorrhea and dysmenorrhea, 141. For suppositories in physometra, 156.

URINE: Urine of an innocent child for washing newborn recommended by some but rejected by Soranus, 82. Rejected as too pungent for exanthemata of children, 122.

VEGETABLES (see also individual names): Vegetables which are not pungent as food in early pregnancy, 47. Most vegetables unsuitable for wet nurse as "watery and not nourishing," 99. As bland food in metasyncritic treatment of chronic amenorrhea and dysmenorrhea, 142.

VINE, WILD: Bloom as astringent for upset stomach in pica, 51. Bloom rejected by Soranus for physometra, 157. Bloom for plasters in hemorrhage of the uterus, 163.

VINEGAR: In remedies for breast to dry up milk, 78. In ointment for skin ulcers of infants, 123. Bread with mixture of oil and vinegar, etc. recommended by some ancients, but rejected by Soranus, in inflammation of the uterus, 148. Asclepiades recommends blowing of vinegar into nose of hysterical patients, 153; Soranus rejects this, 154. In hemorrhage of the uterus, 162; as potion for hemorrhage of the uterus, 162; sitz baths of pure vinegar in hemorrhage of the uterus, 162; for injections in hemorrhage of the uterus, 163; for plasters in hemorrhage of the uterus, 163, 164; with "black remedy" in hemorrhage of the uterus with erosions, 164; in food in hemorrhage of the uterus, 164. Diocles inserts pomegranates dipped in vinegar in prolapse of the uterus, which Soranus rejects, 203.

VINEGAR, DILUTED: As styptic for upset stomach in pica, 51; for preparation of groats of spelt as food in pica, 52; for preparing styptic poultice in painful pica, 52; for preparing easily digestible dish in pica, 52. Applied as astringent in threatening inflammation of

* According to Dioscorides v, 6, 4 (vol. 3, p. 6) the "so-called Cretan wine" is made from dried grapes.

during pregnancy after pica, 55. Diluted wine and abortifacient medication, 65; little wine before bathing promotes abortion, 66; yet abstinence recommended for inducing it, 67. In ointment for breasts to dry up milk, 78. Wine for washing newborn, rejected by Soranus, 82. For wet nurse when the infant has become strong, 100; a little wine for wet nurse if milk is too thin, 103. Crumbs of bread softened in sweet wine for older babies, 117; a little watery wine as drink for babies, 117; diluted wine into which soft bread is dipped as baby drink, 118. Sweet wine for preparation of suppositories in amenorrhea and dysmenorrhea, 140; as restorative treatment in amenorrhea and dysmenorrhea, 141; forbidden on each first day of a new phase in the metasyncritic treatment of amenorrhea and dysmenorrhea, 142. Tart and watery for inflammation of the uterus, 147. In abating hysteria, 152; diluted wine rejected in hysteria when metasyncrisis not desired, 154. Tart wine rejected by Soranus for physometra, 157. In mole during remissions, 160. Tart wine used in plasters for hemorrhage of the uterus, 163; sweet wine for suppositories for hemorrhage of the uterus, 164; dry dregs in suppositories for hemorrhage of the uterus, 164; in abating hemorrhage of the uterus, 164. Tart wine in flux of women, 167; wine in moderation in chronic flux of women, 168. Tart wine externally in gonorrhea, 169; little dry wine as drink in gonorrhea, 169. Moderately dry, astringent in atony of the uterus, 172. For diluting juice of hypocist in prolapse of the uterus, 205; astringent wine externally on wool in prolapse of the uterus, 205; sitz bath in dark tart wine for prolapse of the uterus, 205.

WORMWOOD (*artemisia*): In abortifacient, 66. In sitz bath for physometra, 156. In sitz baths, etc. for mole during remissions, 160; steaming rejected in mole, 161. Fumigations and fomentations in retention of secundines rejected by Soranus, 197 f.

INDEX OF PERSONAL NAMES AND SUBJECTS *

* Drugs and foods discussed by Soranus in his *Gynecology* are listed in the Materia Medica, pp. 215–244.

Printed in the USA
CPSIA information can be obtained
at www.ICGtesting.com
JSHW022158020224
56335JS00004B/14

9 780801 843204